PHOTOINDUCED
PHASE TRANSITIONS

editor

K. NASU
High Energy Accelerator Research Organization (KEK), Japan

World Scientific

NEW JERSEY • LONDON • SINGAPORE • BEIJING • SHANGHAI • HONG KONG • TAIPEI • CHENNAI

Published by

World Scientific Publishing Co. Pte. Ltd.
5 Toh Tuck Link, Singapore 596224
USA office: 27 Warren Street, Suite 401–402, Hackensack, NJ 07601
UK office: 57 Shelton Street, Covent Garden, London WC2H 9HE

British Library Cataloguing-in-Publication Data
A catalogue record for this book is available from the British Library.

PHOTOINDUCED PHASE TRANSITIONS

ISBN 981-238-763-3

Printed in Singapore by World Scientific Printers (S) Pte Ltd

HEALTH PLANNING IN INDIA

HEALTH PLANNING IN INDIA

Edited By
PROF. G. RAMACHANDRUDU
Professor of Economics and Honorary Director
Population Research Centre, Andhra University
Visakhapatnam-530003

A.P.H. PUBLISHING CORPORATION
5, ANSARI ROAD, DARYA GANJ
NEW DELHI - 110 002

Published by

S. B. Nangia
A.P.H. Publishing Corporation
5, Ansari Road, Darya Ganj
New Delhi-110 002
☎ 3274050

ISBN 81-7024-876-0

1997

Typeset at
NEW APCON
25/2, Panchsheel Shopping Centre
New Delhi 110 017
☎ 6460802

Printed in India at
Efficient Offset Printers
New Delhi-110 035

Dedicated to
Bhagawan Sri Sathya Sai Baba
Prasanthi Nilayam
Puttaparthy (A.P.)

Who showed to the world that health care and education should be free to all

INTRODUCTION

Ever since India opted for a planned development approach as far back as in 1951, sectoral planning gained importance, of course, with priority being given to agriculture, industry and infrastructure over social sectors like Health and Education. Probably this trend resulted in the 'Population Explosion' and poor show on the front of Human Development in India (UNDP, 1994). Economists, who are the dominating technocrats in the Planning Commission never envisaged population as an endogenous variable, which probably resulted in the 'missing millions' of people in the planning process over the last five decades.

This book is concerned primarily with the state of health planning in India, as seen in terms of Plan allocations and resulting in different indices of health status of the people and its determinants with special focus on the state of Andhra Pradesh. In a country where nearly a billion people live, out of whom the poor constitutes about one third, substantial plan allocations to health and family planning are very essential. The first paper in the volume by Prof. G. Ramachandrudu and Dr. (Mrs.) G. Kamalamma critically analyses the trends in the plan allocations and health policy. The authors observed that the real per capita expenditure on health have declined during 1955-56 and 1976-77, while the expenditure on family planning has been steeply increasing. They pointed out that without reducing infant mortality through health inventions, mere spending on family planning programme would not yield the expected result of fertility decline to the replacement level. The paper recommend the involvement of private sector including the so called 'fake doctors' whose services are predominantly used in the rural areas, in delivering primary health care services.

M. K. Premi in his paper analyzed the priorities in the health care delivery system. He pointed out that some of the obstacles impeding the speed of concerted implementation of health care programmes are (i) constraints regarding finances

(ii) compartmentalisation in activities in respect of inter-sectoral and intrasectoral coordination (iii) inadequacy of information system and institution of timely corrective measures; and (iv) inadequate community participation. The author was very critical of providing basic minimum services to the rural poor particularly drinking water, sanitation and primary health care. In PHCs many times the necessary drugs are not available even paramedical persons are not found when there was an emergency. He suggested that there has to be increased community and voluntary agencies involvement on the one hand and building of confidence in the government run system on the other.

Fathima Kutty analyzed how green revolution can promote health. She has suggested that it was possible to import green revolution in rural areas to urban areas. She quoted the example of Bandra's Carter Road, Breach Candy and Napean Sea Road in Bombay. It not only prevents disease but also fights against pollution.

K. S. Chalam and D. Francis stressed the importance of health in labour productivity and entrepreneurial ability. They have developed human resource development index of health. It is weighted index of health taking two variables viz. Number of Hospital beds and Doctors in Andhra Pradesh. They have made district-wise analysis. They pointed out that the human resources development index of health shows a declining trend in the formation of health facilities over the period. This was due to increase in population and the norms of bed-patient ratio set by the government. Telangana region is found to be better placed in the formation of human resources development of health.

G. Ramachandrudu and G. Venkata Rao examined the interdistrict variations in Health Services in Andhra Pradesh. The authors pointed out that there are wide inter-district variations in the health infrastructure improvement. The more urbanised districts like Hyderabad and Visakhapatnam have been doing better than the districts with more rural populations. While analysing the inter-district variations, they observed that the variations with regard to the hospitals and dispensaries is increasing whereas the variations in the number of beds available and the number of doctors is decreasing. The study concluded that the health infrastructure is closely related to the Couple Protection Rate (CPR) and hence it recommended that the variation in health infrastructure among districts has to be reduced for the success of family welfare programmes.

P.V.S. Sarma analyzed the demographic implications of the goals of 'Health for All by 2000 A.D.' He observed that though mortality is falling, morbidity is increasing whereas correspondingly health care services are not improving. It is not the question of quantity, what is more important in health is quality. Unless drastic steps are taken to improve the quality of health care delivery system, it would be very difficult to achieve significant reductions in infant mortality rate and maternal mortality rate. He identified that poverty and food scarcity are the basic problems hampering the improvement of health status of the people. Thus he suggested that attack on poverty and controlling population growth are the twin approaches to achieve the goal of health for all.

G. Rama Rao in his paper traces the evolution of health policy in India. He identifies certain demographic variables that hamper the efforts of improving public health and medical care. He pointed out that in addition to the Universal Immunisation Programme, the supply of safe drinking water to rural areas also brought down infant and child mortality at a faster rate. He observed that the gap between rural and urban areas were more among the underdeveloped states such as Uttar Pradesh, Bihar, Madhya Pradesh and Rajasthan, on the other hand, the gap was narrowed among the developed states such as Kerala and Tamil Nadu. He recommended that the primary health care services in the rural areas must substantially be improved.

G. Ramachandrudu critically analysed the mortality and morbidity data sources in India. Though the data on mortality is relatively better, thanks to the persistent improvements, taking place in SRS, the morbidity data collection is still a non-starter. Leave alone state-wise data, even the national level data on morbidity is not systematically collected and analyzed. He has shown with the available data on mortality and morbidity how inadequate is the information. The observation that the still birth rate is higher in urban areas than in the rural areas has to be carefully interpreted. The study pointed out that the prevalence of ARI, Diphtheria and Diarrhoea is very high in Andhra Pradesh, which requires immediate attention of the government.

P. Durga Prasad has clearly brought out the focus on the health status in India by pointing out the inadequate progress with regard to infant and maternal mortality, malnutrition, drinking water, family planning practices, immunisation, incidence of leprosy, T. B., blindness, malaria, goitre, worm infestations, skin infections and other health problem continue to cause disability, panic and death among millions. He highlighted the social and cultural barriers to the improvement of health status of Indian masses. He suggested that the health interventions in rural areas should keep in mind the negative and positive aspects of socio-cultural practices of food, reproduction and health care.

Sriranjani Subba Rao has examined the health problems of the slum dwellers in the city of Visakhapatnam. She observed that about 25 per cent of the city population live in 170 slums and squatter settlements in Visakhapatnam, where migrated labour live with low wage income. Poverty, ignorance and disease are the result of their gloomy future. She pointed out that though there are big government hospitals, slum dwellers very often approach quacks (unqualified doctors) or medical shops to get primary treatment and temporary relief. This inadequate treatment leads to chronic diseases that keeps them out of their jobs resulting in the shattering of the family. Creating community awareness about their environment, special programmes for women and children, encouraging voluntary initiatives for providing health care are some of the recommendations of the author for improving health status of slum dwellers.

G. Parthasarthy critically analyzed the role of the society, particularly of the elite class towards the health of the poor and disadvantaged sections. It is also in the self interest of the elite group since health of poor man has externalities which affect the whole community. He pointed out that there are unhealthy and growing trends of individualism, privatisation, competitive acquisition and consumerism cutting at the root of the ethical base of the society. He strongly pleaded for improving status of women for promoting better health in the family and in the society. This requires a very strong social movement by youth with vision, dedication and commitment.

K. Ranigopal in her paper pointed out that health is an important component of human capital which plays a dominant role in economic development. Neglect of health care is perhaps the most important reason for our low status in the Human Development Index of the UNDP. The most important reason for our low health status is high morbidity. High rural-urban differentials in nutrition, sanitation and drinking water, poor quality of primary health care services, lack of proper referral services are the factors that contribute to the high morbidity. Improvement of the health infrastructure on one side and improving socio-economic status of the people on the other side are two approaches for achieving the goal of Health For All by 2000 A.D.

K. Viswanatham highlighted the importance of education and age at marriage in the improvement of health status of the people. Illiteracy, religion, superstition, and government apathy towards social issues are leading to the atrocity of low age at marriage of girls. Unless the girl attains the age of 21 years, she would not be able to decide what to do, how to do and how many number of children she should have. He was of the view that population problem should be solved for achieving the goal of health for all. He suggested that the differential family planning incentives between employees and non-employees should be removed. Financial incentives for girls marrying at the age of 21 years should be sanctioned and compulsory residential school education for all girls is recommended.

M. Chandrasekhar observed that health is a total concept which includes preventive, promotive, curative and rehabilitative. Health is the responsibility not only of the government, but also the private, non-governmental organisations and more so of every individual. Health care management in India has failed to create adequate health facilities in rural areas inspite of the increasing plan allocations. Growing inequalities in the quality of health care between private and government hospitals is the cause of concern. The cost of health care is enormously increasing. The author suggested policy aspects like collection of user charges in government hospitals, promoting health insurance scheme and improving health information system which are the top priorities for better health management system in India.

K. Kondala Rao is of the view that providing health care at an affordable cost should be the criteria for achieving the goal of health for all. Immunisation programme is the most important cost-effective method of disease control. The UNICEF, ODA, UNPF are generous in sending the materials to the developing countries for conducting immunisation sessions. He observed that preventive aspects of health care should be given priority over curative aspects.

K. Mahadevan and M. Ubaidullah have compared the health programmes in India and Malaysia. While Malaysia spends about 25 per cent of their budget of health, India spends about 5 to 7 per cent for health and family planning programmes in India. They observed that there is a gross under utilisation of public health infrastructure in India because of poor management and supervision. They suggested that the staff at the PHCs should be adequately trained in human relations, medical colleges should adopt one district, improvement of roads and telecommunications in rural areas, and compulsory population education to students. Of all, the most important aspects of health planning is a realistic increase in budget allocation for health Sector in India.

Thus the researchers feel that the most important determinant of the Health Status in India is high population pressure, which has to be solved first. The growing menace of privatisation in Health Sector escalated cost of medical care, which is out of reach of the poor and middle income groups. Public sector appears to have failed even in health care despite enormous investments. The only solution appears to be the promotion of the Health Insurance Scheme (HIS), for which government pays the premiums of the poor.

Dr. G. Ramachandrudu

CONTENTS

PREFACE

Health can not be produced and distributed to the people just like food, clothing and shelter but has to be actively acquired and low. Hence health planning becomes difficult. If planning is for growth, health planning might be construed as growth of health care facilities. In developing countries, mere increase in health care services do not serve any purpose and become a waste, unless people are aware of their own health and its determinants. This is the reason why the most important component of primary health care is 'Health Education' which has to be imparted to the illiterate and innocent masses. This book addresses some of the key social and economic issues in health planning and policy.

Organisation of a Seminar now-a-days has become a tougher proposition in India, since funding for seminars has declined considerably. The second most important problem is to get right people for the right topic. We could solve both these problems in organising the Seminar in the Andhra University Campus, Visakhapatnam with the funding from the University Grants Commission, New Delhi and the University Administration. The participants are eminent personalities from Academics, health administrators and professionals. This book is the result of the Seminar deliberations. All the paper writers have done wonderfully well in revising the papers and brought them in printing format.

Publication of the book is possible through the grant from the 'School of Economics' vide reference No. SOE/SAP III/Pub./94-95.

(Prof. G. Ramachandrudu)

SECTION A

HEALTH PLANNING AND HUMAN RESOURCE DEVELOPMENT

1

HEALTH PLANNING IN INDIA—A CRITICAL EVALUATION

Prof. G. Ramachandrudu and Dr. (Mrs.) G. Kamalamma

INTRODUCTION

During the last four decades or so, there had been a sharp decline in the death rates in many parts of the World, including India. This decline was brought about largely by advances in therapeutic and preventive medicine rather than by any significant rise in the standard of living. With the present knowledge of medicine and public health, it has been possible to effectively neutralise the environment to some extent.

The evolution of a health policy is more or less exogenous to either an economic progress or political turmoil or social reforms. In our efforts to follow the planned development, health policy always envisages to achieve a balance between the gigantic target group of people and very meagre resources to be spent on the health programmes.

In this paper, the historical evolution of India's health policy has been critically reviewed.

HEALTH POLICY AND FIVE YEAR PLANS

It may be seen ridiculous to think of drawing health policy from the drafts of Five Year Plans. Economic Planning in India has essentially meant allocation under heads: hospitals and dispensaries, medical education and research, control of communicable diseases, rural health programmes, training programmes, environmental sanitation, water supply, indigenous system of medicine and homeopathy. Family Planning has been separated from the health sector. Health planning in the successive Five Year Plans has meant varying increases in allocations under these separate heads. In the absence of health planning, free market system permit vast linear expansion of curative services in urban areas based on specialities and super-specialities at the cost of minimum medical health care in rural areas.

In the *first* Five Year Plan, the noval' idea of Community Development Programme has been launched. A vigorous programme of social orientation of medical education through establishment of departments of preventive and social medicine and launching of the primary health centres have been on the top priority of the Government. In the *second* plan, health planning has not received any special attention except, the existing scheme of primary health centres network has been expanded in order to cover the rural living in different terrains of this vast geographical area. External medical aid to eradicate malaria and small pox has been received during this plan period. In the *third* plan, family planning programme has been introduced as an integral part of health plan in order to educate and persuade the rural people to accept small family norm. The *fourth* plan pushed ahead the family planning programme with utmost vigour by promoting IUD and sterilisation. The sweeping policy change in the family planning programme is that the shift from cafeteria approach to extension approach and then to mass vasectomy camps approach have been tried during the plan. The *fifth* plan had two facets: realizing the failure of coercive methods, health, family planning and nutrition were made a component of the Minimum Needs Programme, and to launch frontal attack on poverty. Development was recognised as the best contraceptive. Declaration of emergency and rigorous pursuance of mass sterilisation camps have made the family planning programmes a laughing stock and the late Health Minister Raj Narain has come forward with the idea of family welfare instead of family planning.

During the *sixth* plan, rural health scheme have been given top priority at the cost of urban superspecialities hospitals. In this plan period, the family planning programme has been greatly expanded the scope and content into family welfare programme with an integrated approach towards family planning, maternal and child health and nutrition. It has been felt that acceptance of fertility control programme cannot be brought about solely through a target oriented clinical approach. Basic changes in attitudes towards this problem are necessary and it can be brought about through a persistent and widespread information, education and communication activities and manipulation of several socio-economic variables apart from the provision of basic health and family welfare service.[1]

HEALTH EXPENDITURE IN FIVE YEAR PLANS

One of the major defects of the data on public expenditure on health is that the vast majority of this expenditure is in the non-plan sector and most of the expenditure by the State Government is in this sector. Barnett's[2] calculations for the year 1975-76 show that 73.2 per cent of total health expenditure was in the non-plan sector. He concluded that "health activity is still at least nominally controlled largely by the states, and therefore any analysis of health expenditure must include the non-plan expenditure". Cassen R.H.[3] has made an estimate of the growth in the per capita expenditure on health from Rs. 1.5 in 1955-56 to Rs. 12 in 1976-77. But if an adjustment is made for the rise in prices and make 1970-71 as the base year, the per capita expenditure on health in real terms has declined during 1970s.

The often quoted data on public expenditure on health are the plan-outlays. Table 1 presents the trends of health plan outlays under various programmes from the First Plan to the Sixth Plan. We observe from the table that while in absolute terms allocations to the health sector increased steadily from Rs. 140 crores in the First Plan to Rs. 3862 crores in the Sixth Plan, whereas the percentage share of health outlays in the total plan outlays, decreased from about 3 per cent in the first and second plan to about 2 per cent in the successive plans.

On the other hand, the share of the family planning programme in plan outlays has increased steadily from 1 per cent in the first two plans to 8 per cent in the third to 25 and 26 per cent in Fourth, Fifth and Sixth Plans.

The most striking factors of the plan outlays is the growth of the allotments to the Minimum Needs Programme (MNP) which was introduced in 1974 to introduce holistic element into health policy, and which represents an attempt to tilt the balance in favour of rural areas, has claimed a substantial share in plan allocations in the Fifth and Sixth Plans. Nearly half of the Health outlays have gone to rural health, rural drinking water, slum improvement and nutrition.

HEALTH SECTOR IN THE SEVENTH PLAN

The increasing recognition to the Family Welfare Programme in successive Five Year Plans has reflected with greater vigour in the Seventh Plan, which says that "Family Welfare occupies an important position in the socio-economic development plans. It plays a crucial role in human resource development and in improving the quality of life if our people. It forms an essential and integral part of the 20 Point Programme which stresses the need for the promotion of "family planning on a voluntary basis as a people's movement".[4]

The long term demographic goal approved by the National Development Council is to reduce the net reproduction rate (NRR) to 1 by the year 1996 for the country as a whole and by 2001 in all the states. The goals set for the year 1990 (the end of the Seventh Plan) include the following achievement.[5]

1. an effective contraceptive prevalence rate of 42 per cent.
2. a crude death rate of 10.4
3. a crude birth rate of 29.1
4. an infant mortality rate of 90

During this Plan period number of documents relating to the family welfare programme have been published. One such documents is Revised Strategy for National Family Welfare Programme.[6]

It explicitly and most appropriately recognises the importance of so-called "Beyond Family Planning" measures which affect the course of fertility, such as age at marriage, and also inhibit the use of contraception, such as female literacy and education, status of women, child survival and development, poverty, old age security and importance of sons. What exactly the family welfare programme can do to change these impediments is by no means clear beyond the fact that family planning is currently integrated with the maternal and child health programme. Moreover a reduction in infant mortality is explicitly included as one of the objectives of the population policy.[7]

THE EIGHTH PLAN (1990-95)

By the time this paper is being written the Draft Approach to the Eighth Five Year Plan prepare by the Planning Commission, headed by Mr. Ramakrishna Hedge has been released at Delhi. The only source on the subject available to us is an article by Moni Nag[8]. He says, "most probably the Commission assumes that the increased emphasis on democratic decentralisation and other changes envisaged in the approach paper (e.g. improvement of education, health and women's status) will contribute sufficiently towards decline in population growth rate by reducing the motivation for large family and improving family planning programme. However, demographic and socio-economic research done so far indicates the need for some basic changes in the family planning programme and for identification of priorities within various development sectors that would expedite the shift towards the small family norms".

Table 2 presents the distribution of public resources to different sectors of socio-economic development.

The resource allocation to family planning has decreased from 2 per cent in fourth plan to 1.8 per cent in seventh plan. Same is the case with health and education. The sectors, which recorded an increase are irrigation and energy.

The internal allocation of resources to different family planning activities in the sixth and seventh plans are compared in Table 3.

There has been a substantial increase of resources allocated to each of the items, although the increase is not uniform. Two items—Services and Supplies, and maternal and child health—accounted for 87 per cent of the resources in the Sixth Plan. During the Seventh Plan, the resources under these two heads combined have been more than doubled in absolute amount, although they only account for 69 per cent of all the resources. A substantial increase is envisioned under training, organisation, the village health guides scheme and area projects. Research and evaluation activities account for less than 1 per cent. While we are not certain about the activities included under each of the items listed in Table 3, a cursory look suggests that these allocations do not reflect any strategic change in the use of about Rs. 22 billion additional resources allocated to the Family Welfare Programme activities in the Seventh Plan. It is interesting to note that no resources are explicitly allocated to experimental approaches to deliver services or to create demand for these services.

Table 1 : Health Plan Outlays under Various Programmes (Rs. in Crores)

Programme	*Ist Plan : 1951-56* Outlay	% of Total	*IInd Plan : 1956-61* Outlay	% of Total	*IIIrd Plan : 1961-66* Outlay	% of Total
1	2	3	4	5	6	7
1. Communicable diseases	23.1	16.5	64.0	28.4	70.5	20.6
2. Primary Health Centres, hospitals, dispensaries etc.	25.0	17.9	36.0	16.0	61.7	18.1
3. Indian System of Medicine	0.4	0.3	4.0	1.8	9.0	2.9
4. Education, Training & Research	21.6	15.4	36.0	16.0	56.3	16.4
5. Family Planning	0.7	0.5	3.0	1.3	27.0	7.9
6. Minimum needs programme						
(a) Rural Health	-	-	-	-	-	-
(b) Rural Water Supply	-	-	-	-	-	-
(c) Environmental Improvement of slums	-	-	-	-	-	-
(d) Nutrition	-	-	-	-	-	-
7. Water Supply and Sanitation	49.0	35.0	76.0	33.8	105.3	30.8
8. Others	20.0	14.4	6.0	2.7	11.2	3.3
9. Total	140.0	100.00	225.0	100.00	341.8	100.00

Programme	4th Plan : 1969-74 Outlay	% of Total	5th Plan : 1974-79 Outlay	% of Total	6th Plan : 1980-85 Outlay	% of Total
1	*2*	*3*	*4*	*5*	*6*	*7*
1. Communicable diseases	127.0	10.7	265.0	13.4	524.0	13.8
2. Primary Health Centres, hospitals, dispensaries etc.	164.8	13.6	132.6	6.7	45.0	1.2
3. Indian System of Medicine	15.3	1.3	25.1	1.2	29.0	0.7
4. Education, Training & Research	98.2	8.2	111.2	5.6	62.0	1.6
5. Family Planning	315.0	26.0	497.4	25.1	1010.0	26.1
6. Minimum needs programme						
(a) Rural Health	-	-	140.0	7.0	408.0	10.6
(b) Rural Water Supply	-	-	583.0	29.5	1407.1	36.4
(c) Environmental Impovement of slums	-	-	74.0	3.7	151.5	3.9
(d) Nutrition	45.8	3.8	121.0	6.1	218.7	5.7
7. Water supply and Sanitation	407.3	34.3	-	-	-	-
8. Others	27.7	2.3	27.3	1.4	7.5	0.2
9. Total	1190.8	100.00	1976.8	100.0	3862.8	100.00

Note : a—a crore is 10 million

Source : Government of India (1977 and 1980 (b)

Table 2 : Percentage Distribution of Public Sector Outlay by Sector of Development in Fourth to Seventh Plans

Sector of Development	*Fourth Plan 1969-74*	*Fifth Plan 1974-79*	*Sixth Plan 1980-85*	*Seventh Plan 1985-90*
1	2	3	*4*	*5*
Economic				
Agriculture and allied sectors[1]	17.1	11.0	12.9	12.7
Irrigation and flood control	6.8	10.7	12.5	9.4
Energy	15.4	26.2	27.2	30.4
Industry and Minerals	22.8	18.7	15.4	12.5
Transport and Communications	20.3	17.6	15.9	16.4
Social				
Education	6.1	3.3	2.6	3.5
Health	2.7	1.7	1.9	1.9
Family Planning[2]	2.0	1.3	1.0	1.8
Others[3]	6.8	9.5	10.6	11.6
Total %	100.00	100.00	100.00	100.00
Public Sector outlay (in million Rs.)	159,020	393,220	975,000	1,800,000

1. Includes agriculture, allies areas, and rural development
2. Includes maternal and child health
3. Others includes science and technology; other social services including water and sanitation, social and women's welfare, nutrition, housing and urban development; and others.

Table 3 : Allocation of Family Planning* Resources in Sixth and Seventh Plans

Programme	*Outlay in Million Rs.*			*Percent Distribution of plan outlay*	
	Sixth Plan	*Seventh Plan*	*Ratio 2 ÷ 1*	*Sixth Plan*	*Seventh Plan*
	1	*2*	*3*	*4*	*5*
1. Services and Supplies	6877	13569	1.97	63.8	41.7
2. Training	88	609	6.92	0.8	1.9
3. Research and Evaluation	115	250	2.17	1.1	0.8
4. Indian Council of Medical Research	-	500	N.A.	-	1.5
5. Mass Media & Education	320	1050	3.28	3.0	3.2
6. Maternal & Child Health	2503	8885	3.55	23.2	27.3
7. Organization	195	1250	6.41	1.8	3.8
8. Village Health Guides Scheme	680	3700	5.44	6.3	11.4
9. Area Projects	-	2750	NA	-	8.4
10. Indian Population Projects	2	-	NA	**	-
Total	10780	32563	3.02	100.00	100.00

* Includes Maternal and Child Health.

** Less than 0.1 per cent

— Not available, NA = Not applicable; Source : Sixth Five Year Plan p. 385, Seventh Five Year Plan pp. 281 and 291.

SOCIAL AND ECONOMIC DIMENSIONS OF HEALTH POLICY

"Health has been defined as a state of complete physical, mental and social well being and not mere absence of disease or infirmity"[9] This is a very broad concept of health and implies a perfect harmony of the internal environment of man and the external environment consisting of physical, chemical and biological sorroundings. Unfortunately, health cannot be given or distributed, but has to be actively acquired and won.

As man is inseparable from Nature it is not surprising that the environment in which man lives, has a profound influence on him, in spite of his magnificent achievements in becoming the master of the world. All the living organisms, including man, live in a highly competitive struggle for survival, Man's internal environment, therefore, is constantly under the influence of the external forces of nature.

Existing literature on health policy is concentrated around the set goals and how to achieve them by plan allocations, or expansion of health services. Beyond these plan instruments, there are certain cultural, social and economic dimensions of health policy, which are often ignored or assumed away. For example, there are three major indigenous systems of medicine in India : Ayurveda—the Hindu Medical System; Unani the Greek System of medicine which was brought to India from West Asia by the Muslim rulers of India; and the Siddha System, which was considered to be a specialised branch of Ayurveda. The British rule in India has practically destroyed these three medical systems and imported the Allopathic system, the western medical care, and later Indian leaders also have not paid much attention to these original Indian hereditary schools of medicine, as such there is a sharp deterioration in the body of knowledge, in their instructions for training and research, in the drug industry, and in their corps of practitioners.

Even today we see here and there, the old people in the villages, giving herbs or other medicines for free of cost and people trusting them as a source of medical facility as the first step. In majority of the villages, now the "Quack doctors", calling themselves as the "Registered Medical Practitioners", are minting money out of ignorance of the rural people and easy availability of these services make the people to approach them. Even though there is a wide criticism against these doctors, Government seem to be not contemplating any corrective action against these quack doctors.

Any writing on health policy without reference to the health goals of "Health for All By 2000 AD" would be considered incomplete, because the resolutions adopted by 134 members countries of World Health Organisation assembled at Alma Ata, USSR, during 6-12 September, 1978, are so vital to the health policy, especially the primary health care. "Human resources of a country are undoubtedly the most precious endowment. Health care is intrinsic to the well being of the people and has to be promoted as an economic value, and as a means to reduce absenteeism, bedility, disability, and raise efficiency, productivity and finally the income earning capacity. These aspects of the goal have certain implications to the Indian economy. The health status of the millions of people in the world today causes considerable concern, and the story of the developing countries is particularly pathetic. On the global level, it calls for a new approach to close the gap between 'haves' and 'have nots' through equitable distribution of health resources, transfer of health technologies, upgradation of skills and information systems, strengthening of infrastructure so as to ensure the level of health for all the citizens of the world, and enable them lead a socially meaningful and economically productive life. It is in this context the concept of primary health care, i.e. access for all to minimum health care, close to their homes, so as to enable all people lead a healthy life, is stressed."[10]

In spite of several efforts on the part of the Government, the health care programmes are not reaching fully to the ultimate consumers. It is observed that only 10 to 20 per cent of the population are utilising Government Health Programmes and the rest of the population prefer either home remedies or private medical practioners.[11]

Siva Raju[12] writes, "primary health care includes many components like, community participation, social structure, physical factors, availability of technological tools, indigenous health practices, and linkages between new and old technological systems for curative and preventive health services in the community. As delivery of health care is to reach everyone throughout the country, there exists a necessity for optimum integration of various components of health care system depending on the socio-economic and cultural background of each community. In this regard, comprehensive evaluative studies on the existing patterns of health care services by taking into consideration the various components of primary health care like, government health programmes, role of private medical practitioners, etc.

HEALTH TRANSITION IN INDIA AND ANDHRA PRADESH

Mortality and morbidity, even though both seem to be the two faces of the same coin, they differ very widely in terms of their levels, trends and determinants. For example Kerala State in India has one of the lowest mortality levels among all States, but yet morbidity is reported to be highest in the State. The plausible reasons may be the higher proportion of old people in the State, better statistical reporting system and greater health awareness of people.

Table 4 presents trends of All India Rural mortality rates during 1976-84. Crude death rate has declined from 16.3 in 1976 to 13.8 in 1984. Infant mortality rate has declined from 139 in 1976 to 113.3 in 1984. Neo-natal mortality rate has been reduced from 83 in 1976 to 72.2 in 1984. Post-natal mortality rate has been reduced from 56 in 1976 to 41.1 in 1984. Pre-natal mortality rate has been reduced from 76 7 in 1976 to 58.3 in 1984. Lastly still birth rate has been reduced from 18.7 in 1976 to 11 in 1984. Of all the decline in mortality rates decline in the infant mortality rate has been striking and significant.

Table 5 presents the trends of infant mortality rates of Andhra Pradesh and All India and for rural and urban areas separately. In Andhra Pradesh, rural infant mortality rate has declined from 136 in 1977 to 81 in 1984, but there is slight rise to 90 in 1985. Urban infant mortality rate, however, declined to the lowest from 97 in 1976 to 40 in 1980, but it shot up to 66 in 1984 and again it has been recorded a fall to 57 in 1985.

Similarly All India rural infant mortality rate has declined from 140 in 1977 to 107 in 1985. The decline was consistent. Urban infant mortality rate has also recorded a steep fall from 81 in 1977 to 59 in 1985.

ACHIEVEMENT OF HEALTH GOALS

Table 6 presents the classification of States/Union territories according to coverage of population by sub-centre. Out of 31 States/

Table 4 : Rural Mortality Indicators (1976-84) All India

Year	*Crude Death Rate*	*Infant Mortality Rate*	*Neo-Natal Mortality Rate*	*Post-Natal Mortality Rate*	*Peri-Natal Mortality Rate*	*Still Birth Rate*
1	2	*3*	*4*	*5*	*6*	*7*
1976	16.3	139.0	83.0	56.0	76.6	18.7
1977	16.0	140.0	88.0	52.0	69.5	16.8
1978	15.3	137.0	85.2	51.8	67.9	16.0
1979	13.9	129.7	77.7	52.0	63.1	13.3
1980	13.5	123.8	75.5	48.3	59.8	12.0
1981	13.7	119.1	75.5	48.3	58.8	11.4
1982	13.1	113.7	72.9	40.8	57.7	9.8
1983	13.1	113.8	73.6	40.2	57.7	9.4
1984	13.8	113.3	72.2	41.1	58.3	11.0
1985	13.0	107.0	66.6	39.9	52.4	10.8
1986	12.2	105.0	65.5	39.1	51.8	10.5
1987	12.0	104.0	63.6	40.5	54.4	13.6
1988	12.0	102.0	62.0	40.1	53.1	13.9
1989	11.1	98.0	-	-	-	-
1990	10.1	86.0	-	-	-	-

Source : Year Book 1990-91, Family Welfare Programme in India, Department of Family Welfare, Ministry of Health and Family Welfare, Government of India.

Union territories only 17 States/Union territories falling in the population ranges, less than 3000 and 3000-5000 have achieved the National Norm of population to be served by a sub-centre. Our National Norm for sub-centre is that every 3000-5000 population there must be a sub-centre. In Andhra Pradesh there is a sub-centre for every 5684 people. This far away from the National Norm. In our country 14 States/Union territories did not achieve the National Norm.

Table 5 : Infant Mortality Rate (1976 to 85) Andhra Pradesh and All India

Year	*Andhra Pradesh*		*All India**	
	Rural	*Urban*	*Rural*	*Urban*
1976	127	97	139	80
1977	136	62	140	81
1978	127	66	137	74
1979	114	65	130	72
1980	103	40	124	65
1981	93	52	119	62
1982	86	50	114	65
1983	83	54	114	66
1984	81	66	113	66
1985	90	57	107	59
1986	87	59	105	62
1987	84	58	104	61
1988	89	63	102	62
1989	88	53	98	58
1990	73	56	86	51

* The aggregate estimates form All India from 1976 to 1980 exclude Bihar and West Bengal.

Source : Same as table 4.

Table 6 : Classification of States/Union Territories According to Coverage of Population by A.P.H.C.

Sl. No.	*Range of Population*	*No. of States/ U.T.S. in the Rate*	*States/U.T.S. having achieved the Population Range*	
1	*2*	*3*	*4*	
1.	<10000	2	1. Lakshadweep (3429)	2. Punjab (7090)
2.	10000-20000	4	3. A & N Islands (14161)	4. Mizoram (14348)
			5. Sikkim (16035)	6. Pondicherry (16339)
3.	20000-30000	6	7. Jammu & Kashmir (20860)	8. Meghalaya (23483)
			9. Manipur (24412)	10. Himachal Pradesh (27960)
			11. Maharashtra (29070)	12. D & N Haveli (28925)
4.	30000-40000	7	13. Nagaland (30085)	14. West Bengal (31971)
			15. Andhra Pradesh (34973)	16. Arunachal Pradesh (35075)
			17. Orissa (35473)	18. Haryana (37914)
			19. Kerala (38298)	
5.	40000-50000	7	20. Uttar Pradesh (40659)	21. Gujarat (41180)
			22. Tamil Nadu (42084)	23. Goa* (43078)
			24. Tripura (43920)	25. Bihar (44851)
			26. Madhya Pradesh (44747)	
6.	50000 & above	4	27. Rajasthan (52524)	28. Assam (52675)
			29. Karnataka (53082)	30. Delhi (56782)

Note : Chandigarh has not established by P.H.C. * include the information of Daman & Diu Figures are provisional.

Table 7 represents the classification of States/Union territories according to coverage of population by a Primary Health Centre. According to our National Norm 20000-30000 population to be served by a primary health centre. Out of 31 States/Union territories 12 States/ Union territories falling in the three ranges less than 10000, 10000-20000 and 20000-30000 have achieved the National Norm of population to be served by the primary Health Centre.

For primary health centres also Andhra Pradesh did not achieve the National Norm. Apart from Andhra Pradesh the remaining 17 States did not achieve the National Norm. In Andhra Pradesh 34,973 people were served by a primary health centre.

Table 8 presents the classification of States/Union territories according to coverage of population by a community health centre. According to our National Norm about one lakh population to be served by a community health centre. Out of 31 States/Union territories 28 States/Union territories have established community health centres. Sikkim, Dadar and Nagar Haveli and Delhi have not established any community health centres. Out of 28 States/Union territories which have community health centres only Chandigarh and Lakshadweep have achieved the National Norm population to be served by a community health centre. In Andhra Pradesh there is a C.H.C. for every 9.75 lakh population. This is far away from the National Norm (about one lakh).

Table 9 presents the gap between the set of national norms (goals) and their achievement as on 30.9.1988. Out of 16 health indicators, goals are set for 10 indicators, and all the 10 indicators, except one, are far beyond the targeted goal, the set goal for the ratio of HA (M) : HW (M) was 1:6, but the actual achievement of the ratio is 1:35.

The achievement of the goal of health for all depends primarily on the expansion and optimum utilisation of health services. If the provision of health facilities is the necessary condition for achieving the goal of Health for all, people's participation in utilising the services in an optimal ways is the sufficient condition. That is the reason why, probably, the World Health Organisation (WHO) has modified the slogan of "Health for All by 2000 AD" to "Health for All and All for Health by 2000 AD". Without effective demand for health services,

Table 7 : Classification of States/Union Territories According to Coverage of Population by a Sub-Centre

Sl. No.	*Range of Population*	*No. of States/ U.T.S. in the Range*	*States/U.T.S. having achieved the Population Range*	
1	*2*	*3*	*4*	
1.	Less than 3000	4	1. Lakshadweep (1714)	2. Mizoram (2263)
			3. Sikkim (2607)	4. Chandigarh (2625)
2.	3000-5000	13	5. Manipur (3013)	6. Andaman & Nicobar Islands (3068)
			7. Jammu Kashmir (3906)	8. Himachal Pradesh (3998)
			9. Pondicherry (4028)	10. Nagaland (4041)
			11. Gujarat (4127)	12. Meghalaya (4185)
			13. D & N Haveli (4285)	14. Tamil Nadu (4580)
			15. Punjab (4780)	16. Maharashtra (4843)
			17. Uttar Pradesh (4994)	
3.	5000-7000	13	18. Karnataka (5063)	19. Madhya Pradesh (5190)
			20. Orissa (5270)	21. Goa (5282)
			22. Arunachal Pradesh (5684)	23. Haryana (5404)
			24. Andhra Pradesh (5684)	25. West Bengal (5867)
			26. Kerala (5882)	27. Tripura (6114)
			28. Assam (6362)	29. Rajasthan (6554)
			30. Bihar (6635)	
4.	7000 & Above	1	31. Delhi (10811)	

Figures are Provisional

Table 8 : Classification of States/Union Territories According to Coverage of Population by a Health Centre

Sl. No.	*Range of Population*	*No. of States/ U.T.S. in the Rate*	*States/U.T.S. having achieved the Population Range*	
1	2	3	4	
1.	Less than 3	15	1. Lakshadweep (0.24)	2. Chandigarh (0.31)
			3. Mizoram (1.11)	4. Arunachal Pradesh (1.40)
			5. Himachal Pradesh (1.40)	6. Manipur (1.49)
			7. Maharashtra 1.61)	8. Andaman & Nicobar Islands (1.84)
			9. J & K (1.99)	10. Goa* (2.05)
			11. Gujarat (2.69)	12. Nagaland (2.70)
			13. Tripura (2.70)	14. Karnataka (2.75)
			15. Pondicherry (2.94)	
2.	3-5	8	16. Punjab (3.00)	17. Orissa (3.06)
			18. Haryana (3.60)	19. Rajasthan (3.65)
			20. Madhya Pradesh (4.02)	21. Meghalaya (4.22)
			22. Assam (4.82)	23. Tamil Nadu (4.90)
3.	5-7	2	24. West Bengal (5.56)	25. UP (6.99
4.	7 and above	3	26. Kerala (7.85)	27. Bihar (9.00)
			28. Andhra Pradesh (9.75)	

Note : 1. Sikkim, D & N Haveli and Delhi have not established any community health centres.
2 Figures in brackets indicate population in lakhs
* include the information of Daman & Diu. (Figures are provisional)

Table 9 : Level of Achievement of some norms all India Position as on 30-9-1938

S. No.	*Parameters/Indicators*	*National Norms*	*Norms achieved/ Established (Approximate)*
1	2	3	*4*
1.	Population covered by a sub-centre	3000-5000 Pop	5304
2.	Population covered by a PHC	20000-30000	35371
3.	Population covered by a Community Health Centre	About 1 lakh Pop	4.07 lakhs
4.	No. of sub-centres for each PHC	6 sub-centres	6.7 sub-centres
5.	No. of Primary health centres for each Community Health Centre	4 PHCs	11.5 PHCs
6.	Trained village Health guide	One for each village/ 1000 Population	1.44 villages/ 1331 Population
7.	Trained Dai	Atleast one for each village	1.03 villages (1029 population)
8.	Population served by health workers (Male and Female)	Male 3000-5000 Female 3000-5000	7188 5261
9.	Ratio of HA (M) : HW (M)	1:6	1:3.5
10.	Ratio of HA (F) : HW (F)	1:6	1:6.3

S. No.	*Parameters/Indicators*	*National Norms*	*Norms achieved/ Established (Approximate)*
1	2	3	*4*
11.	Average area covered by a sub-centres	-	28.50 sq. km.
12.	Average area covered by a PHC	-	190.09 sq. km.
13.	Average area covered by a CHC	-	2190.41 sq. km.
14.	Max. Radial distance covered by a sub-centre (in km.)	-	3.01
15.	Max. radial distance covered by a PHC (in km.)	-	7.78
16.	Max. radial distance covered by a CHC (in khm.)	-	26.40

mere supply of them would become a waste.

The backbone of rural health programme is the primary health centre and its vast net work of sub-centres. Studies on strengthening such primary health centres, are not many and there is an urgent need for analysing the problems and their solutions of the rural health services. Generally problems range from non-availability of medical personal, medicines to non-response of public in matters relating to the Government sponsored health schemes like immunisation, mother and child health, nutrition programme, etc. Thus, role of voluntary organisations and political commitment on the part of the Government are generally recommended in such situations.

THE GIGANTIC TASK

The health survey and development committee[13] which was set up by the British Indian Government in 1943 to draw a blueprint of health services for the post-war British India, had shown exceptional vision and courage to make some very bold recommendations. These included development of an elaborate health service system for the country, giving key importance to preventive aspects with "the country side as the focal point"[14]. To forestall any criticism of practicability, pointing out the achievements in health in the Soviet Union within a span of 28 years (1913-1941) it asserted that its recommendations are quite practical, infect relatively very modest provided there was the will to develop the health services of the country.[15] Unfortunately, however, the leaders who took over from the British did not show this will. In turn the health policy in India has led the country of wide and growing rural-urban disparities in the health services, destroying the native medicare systems. Relatively free enterprise medical systems in India, the poor are exploited the maximum and access to modern medicine has been limited by the price of health services, which is kept high. Under these circumstances, people are naturally tended towards the cheap, and easily accessible quack doctors available in the villages.

Evolution of any health policy without referring to the existing reality of dominating and popularising Registered Medical Practitioner (Quack doctors) of the rural, semi-urban and even urban areas will be not only unrealistic but also self-defeating. No serious attempt has been made on the concept of "bare-foot doctors" which is initiated during the Janata Regime in 1978. What is now required is to streamline or regulate the services of these RMPs or quack doctors. Every RMP must register their names in taluk hospitals and attend periodic training camps. They must also be authorised to treat certain cases only, which are of first-aid nature. Villages need immediate attention for injuries in accidents, snake or dog bites, diarrhoea and fevers. So, Government must evolve a policy of roping in these RMPs, and see the rural medicare system is not weakened but strengthened by free flow of funds to the rural health sectors, manage the funds properly and evolve a health policy to rope in the organised as well as unorganised private medical sector and voluntary organisations.

In the domestic front, enhancing the women's status should be top priority in the public policy. Female Education and employment are the twin key issues in this regard. Effective implementation of the existing policies on women should be ascertained. Educated mother would be not only a good teacher but also a good doctor at home. Responsibility of the mother has not ended with bringing up children upto the school going age, but it is extended to take special care with regard to adolescent health. In developing countries more than half the population is under 25 years of age. The problems of this age group ranges from early marriage and reproduction, drugs, unwanted pregnancy, sexually transmitted diseases (STDs) and violence. The solution to these problems largely lie in population and their education, proper implementation of youth policy, and eradication of illiteracy and unemployment.

REFERENCES

1. Banarji, D. "Health and Population Control in the Draft Plan", *Economic and Political Weekly,* Special Number, August, 1979.
2. Barnett, A. "an Introduction to the Health Planning and Budgeting Systems in India", Brighten: IDS discussion Paper 121 (1977) quoted in Radhika Ramasubban—The Development of Health Policy in India in *India's Damography—Essays on the Contemporary Population* (ed) by Tim Dyson and N. Crook, South Asian Publishers' Pvt. Ltd. (1984).
3. Cassen, R. H. (1978), India, Population, Economy, Society, Mc Millan (London)
4. Planing Commission, India, 1985, (279)
5. Radhika Rama Subtan : Op. cit.
6. Department of Family Welfare, Government of India, Revised Strategy for National Family Welfare Programme—A Summary", (Year not specified.)
7. The Population Council: Population and Programmes in India,

September, 1987.

8. Moni Nag, Population Programme and the Eighth Plan Need for Some Basic Changes, *Indian Express*, 10th May, 1990.
9. Deodhar N.S.—"The concept of Health and Disease" in you and your Health (eds). V. N. Bhave, N. S. Deodhar, and S. V. Bhave, National Book Trust, India (1983-Reprint)
10. Chandrasekhar, S., Sanjeeva Reddy, P.L., Rani Gopal, K. "Towards 2000 AD : Indian Health Economy and Policy", M/s. Chugh Publications, 1989.
11. Giffith, D.H.S. (1993), Final Report on Public Health Programmes, Andhra Pradesh, WHO Project, India, SEA/PHA/30 and Department of International Health, John Hopkins University (1976)—Functional Analysis of Health Needs and Services", New York, Asia Publishing House.
12. Sivaraju, S., "Health for All By 2000 AD Need for Comprehensive Evaluation", IASP. 13th Annual Conference (1938) contributed papers (p. B-4).
13. Government of India, "Health Survey and Development Committee" (1946), Report, Vol. II, Delhi, Manager of Publications.
14. Ibid.
15. Ibid.

2

SOME ISSUES IN ATTAINING HEALTH FOR ALL

Mahendra K. Premi

With regard to health, the Directive Principle of the Indian Constitution enunciates that "the state shall regard the raising of the level of nutrition and the standard of living of its people and the improvement of public health as among its primary duties" (article 47). Further, the State shall, in particular, direct its policy towards securing : .... that the health and the strength of workers, men and women, and the tender age of children are not abused and that citizens are not forced by economic necessity to enter avocations unsuited to their age or strength ...... that children are given opportunities and facilities to develop in a healthy manner and in conditions of freedom and dignity and that childhood and youth are protected against exploitation and against moral and material abandonment" (article 39). These directive principles were laid down probably recognising the fact that good health also means proper human resources development.

World Health Organisation states that "health, which is a state of complete physical, mental, and social well-being and not merely the absence of disease or infirmity, is a fundamental human right and that the attainment of highest possible level of health is a most important social goal whose realisation requires the action of many other social and economic sectors in addition to health sector."

India is a signatory to the Alma Ata declaration on "Health for All by the Year 2000". Hence the Government of India is committed to take all necessary steps to achieve this goal.

Since health of a society is intimately related to its value system, its philosophical and cultural traditions, and its social, economic and political organisation, it is not possible to raise the health status of a people unless such efforts are integrated with the wider effort to bring about the overall cultural social, economic and political transformation of the society as a whole.

At the time of independence, some of the important indicators of the health status of our people were almost at a shocking level. Moreover, whatever was available, was very much urbanised and localised in big towns and cities. There were also some dispensaries scattered around the districts with a hospital at the district headquarters or at the headquarters of towns/sub-divisions. With the setting up of the Planning Commission in 1950 and with the general acceptance of the recommendations of the Shore Committee, the planning process of social and economic development covered the health sector also with the setting up of rural primary health centres (one for a population of one lakh or so) on the curative side and programmes of eradication and control of various diseases on the preventive side.

Over the post 40-45 years, there has been a significant achievement on various fronts. The crude death rate declined from about 27 per thousand population in 1941-51 to less than 11 in 1988. The infant mortality rate declined from about 160 per thousand live births in 1941-51 to 129 in 1971 and to 94 in 1988. Smallpox with used to take a heavy toll of life and inflict disfiguring morbidity on the population has been wiped out from the country by the mid 1970s. The incidence and prevalence of many communicable diseases has been reduced very substantially. Malaria which used to be responsible for more that 7.5 crore cases per year at the time of independence, accounts for only 20 lakh cases annually today. Deaths due to malaria have declined from an alarming figure of 7.5 lakh per year to around 15000 by 1986.

The health infrastructure in the country has also increased very substantially over the past forty years. As of 31 March, 1987 there have been 16,449 PHCs and subsidiary Health Centres, 109,644 Subscentres, and 1293 Community Health Centres (CHCs) in the country. At the grassroots level. There are 559000 trained birth attendants (dias)—roughly at least one per village on an average, 392,000 village health guides (VHGs), and 85000 male and 108000 female multi-purpose health workers respectively to take the basic health care services to the doorsteps of the people. The total number of medical practitioners is well above 6 lakhs, over half of them pursue the allopathic system of medicine. In addition, there are more than 1.5 lakh nurses and as many midwives, most of them being in the public health care system. As a result of all this, the expectation of life at birth has increased from 32 in 1941-51 to around 55 in 1985-86. On the basis of the progress made so far, one may safely conclude that India will be able to achieve an IMR of about 60, a crude death rate of 9, and a life expectation of 65 years by the end of the present century, that is, the targets laid down in the National Health Policy, 1982 would more or less be achieved.

In spite of all this achievement, the "Approach Paper to the Eight Five Year Plan 1990-95:" says that it will be impossible to achieve "Health for All by the Year 2000" at the current rate of expansion of health services. Besides, a substantial chunk of whatever health services and medical education are available are appropriated by the upper classes. Health delivery systems in rural areas are inadequate and defective.

ISSUES RELATED TO HEALTH FOR ALL

With the above perspective in view, let us examine some of the issues relating to the topic of this Seminar. In the first instance "Health for All" emphasises more on the preventive aspects of medical science and public health engineering rather than so much on curative aspects. The preventive aspects include control and eradication of various diseases, control of factors which lead to poor health, e.g. malnutrition of the mother and the child, poor immunisation, environmental degradation, poor water supply and sanitation, industrial health hazards, prevalence of various diseases particularly in endemic areas, and indifferences of the people towards their own health. In contrast, the curative aspects include further development of medical infrastructure, availability of drugs, doctors, paramedical personnel, etc. not only in the cities and towns but also in the far flung and remote rural areas. I shall now review the situation of these aspects of health in the country.

NUTRITION

Nutritional status of a population, particularly of its children, is a crucial indicator in determining their quality of life. Malnutrition has adverse influence on morbidity, mortality and life expectancy.

In India, where 39.9 per cent people in the rural areas, and 27.7 per cent in the urban areas (1984-85) are below the poverty line, malnutrition, a by product of poverty and unemployment, continues to be a major problem. It is more acute among infants, pre-school children and expectant and nursing mothers from poor socio-economic groups. This is reflected in greater incidence of protein energy malnutrition (PEM), anaemia, night blindness, and goitre in the rural and low SES population. There have been considerable statewise variations in the nutritional status of children. During 1982, Gujarat had the highest proportion of moderately and severely malnourished children (44.4 per cent and 15.2 per cent respectively) while Kerala had the lowest (4.7 per cent in all).

To improve the nutrition of the children and of expectant and lactating mothers, several nutrition intervention programmes like the Integrated Child Development Services, special nutrition programmes, balwadi nutrition programmes, mid-day meal programme, and wheat-based supplementary nutrition programme have been implemented by the Government of India and several other agencies. Around 25 million children and expectant and nursing mothers have been covered by the above nutrition intervention programmes. There have, however, been several snags in the implementation of these schemes for various reasons. Moreover, it would be necessary to extend the programmes to reach children in small and remote villages.

IMMUNISATION STATUS

The Universal Immunisation Programme (UIP) which was started in 1985-86 by covering the earlier "expanded immunisation programme" into it has proved to be the most cost-effective of the health programmes and is vital to our attaining the objective of "Health for All. "The UIP is against six common vaccine-preventable diseases and for expectant mothers against tenancy. The programme aims to cover 85 per cent infants and 100 per cent pregnant women by 1990. The UIP is aimed to reduce neonatal tetanus mortality to less than one per thousand live births from the current estimated level of 13.3 and 3.2 per thousand live births in rural and urban areas respectively. The incidence of polio-myelitis is expected to be brought down to a negligible level by 1990 when it is estimated to vary from 1.5 to 1.7 per 1000 children (of 0-4 years in age) in the urban and 1.6 to 1.8 in the rural areas.

Although immunisation coverage has increased very substantially since 1980-81, based on the report of the UNICEF on the State of the World's Children 1990 as of March 1988 the immunisation coverage of children below one year was 72 per cent against BCG, 73 per cent against DPT (three doses), 64 per cent against polio (3 doses), and 44 per cent against measles. Further, 58% of pregnant women had been immunised against tetanus by administration of two doses of tetanus toxoid. Obviously, there are regional and state level difference in immunisation performance. Poor performing states will have to put lot of additional efforts in the 1990s to achieve universal immunisation of children and pregnant women. This may also involve restructuring of certain nutrition intervention programmes as indicated in the Approach Paper to the Eight Plan.

Recognising the prime importance of the U.I.P. in the overall health plans, a "Technology Mission of Vaccination and Immunisation" of vulnerable population, especially children was recently set up by the Government to reduce morbidity and mortality of infants and children, and to achieve self-sufficiently in vaccine production. Besides extending the coverage under the present immunisation programme and building up the logistic support, the Mission aims to develop a surveillance system, promote community participation, and encourage research and development of new vaccines.

WATER SUPPLY AND SANITATION

Although a national water supply programme was launched in 1954 during the First Five Year Plan itself, and progressively larger allocations were made for water supply and sanitation, the progress made in the provision of safe drinking water supply and basic sanitation has hardly been satisfactory. By March 1980, about 2 lakh villages in the country with a population of around 160 million were yet to be provided with potable water supply facilities. In hundreds of small and medium towns, water supply and sanitation arrangements were far from adequate. Besides hardship and inconvenience to the poor, especially women and children, in areas where water is scarce, inadequate or polluted, there has been colossal wastage of human resources because of morbidity caused by water-borne or water related diseases which constitute nearly 80% of the public health problem of our country.

The United Nations declared the 1980s as the "International Drinking Water Supply and Sanitation Decade". During the Seventh Plan, the aim was to provide adequate drinking water facilities for the total population and to provide sanitation facilities to 80% of the urban and at least 25% of the rural population.

At the beginning of the Sixth Plan, 2.31 lakh villages were identified as problem villages. Out of these, 1.92 lakh villages were provided with at least one source of drinking water during the Sixth Plan. Due to recurring drought in several states, failure of tube-wells owing to lowering of water level etc., the number of problem villages increased from the balance of 39000 at the beginning of the Seventh Plan to 2.29 lakh during this plan itself. By end of 1987, 1.28 lakh villages have been covered by potable water supply.

With a view to tackle the drinking water supply problem in rural areas, a Technology Mission on Drinking Water in villages and Related Water Management was launched by the Govt. of India in August 1986 with the specific objective to cover all residual problem villages by 1990 and to take conservation measures for sustained drinking water supply. To achieve the above objectives, 50 Mini-Missions and 5 Sub-Missions include (i) eradication of guinea worms; (ii) control of flourishes; (iii) removal of iron from drinking water, (iv) desalination of water, and (v) conservation of water and recharging of ground water aquifers. The Eighth Plan will ensure that no village is left without a protected source of drinking water.

As of 31 March 1985, 57 lakh of rural people (merely one per cent could claim to have sanitation; in urban areas one-third of the population was covered. A UNDP assisted survey of 210 towns in 11 states and 3 Union Territories in the early 1980s revealed that 27 per cent of the population had flush latrines, 40% used dry latrines, and 33% made use of open areas in congested urban localities. According to UNDP calculations, even if the Government concentrated exclusively on converting dry latrines into "pour flush" systems, it would take more than 100 years to achieve the target.

In order to improve rural sanitation, the programme was added to the Minimum Needs Programme from 1987-88 and in the 20-Point Programme as a component of "Health for All". The Seventh Plan envisaged to provide sanitation facilities to at least 25% of the rural population to improve the quality of life. The programme can gather momentum only with people's participation and through self-help schemes organised by the village community and large scale mobilisation of voluntary efforts.

In respect of sanitation, besides provision of proper latrines, the major problem relates to the drainage system. Most of the water borne diseases in both rural and urban areas are caused by stagnant water pools and open drainage systems. Much attention has not been paid to this aspect of public health engineering which is as serious as potable water supply and flush or "pour flush" latrines. Unless the Eighth and the Ninth Plan give priority to the improvement of drainage system in both rural and urban areas, "Health for All" will remain a mirage.

ENVIRONMENTAL DEGRADATION AND INDUSTRIAL HEALTH HAZARDS

National Programmes for the promotion of sanitation, public health, nutrition, housing etc., have been launched in the different five year plan periods and accorded sufficiently high priority, but a comprehensive and integrated view of environmental protection and improvement with emphasis on the sustainable use of natural resources did not receive significant attention till recent years. As a result of mass-scale industrialisation programmes, environment is being polluted every day and is endangering the health of the population. Incidence of occupational and industry related diseases is increasing as well as new diseases are arising out of various industrial pollutants. Nobody can forget the Bhopal gas disaster even after five years. There are many hazardous industries in which constant working by the children and women, especially children leads to permanent disability. The Prevention of Child Labour Act, 1987 has prohibited employment of children in hazardous industries but it goes on unabated as there is hardly any check in those industries.

The issues in the field of environment are pollution control (both air and water); environment protection and conservation education and awareness; organisational and regulatory measures for hazardous substances; ecological research; Ganga Action Plan, etc., The Environment (Protection) Act, 1986 has been promulgated with effect from 19 November 1986 for prevention and control of air and water pollution.

To sustain social and economic development, especially in rural areas, steps are necessary to protect the remaining forests and to enhance the biomass resources particularly through development of waterlands. Sustainable management of forests would require an institutional framework to facilitate people's active involvement which can become a part of a larger approach to the local area planning and development.

CONTROL OF COMMUNICABLE AND OTHER DISEASES

The major disease control programmes for communicable and non-communicable diseases are run basically as centrally sponsored schemes. Some of these schemes have been in operation for almost four decades. As indicated earlier, deaths due to malaria have come down sharply but can further be reduced. Diarrhoea diseases are a major health problem in India especially among children below five years of age. While the cases seeking medical care in the existing health facilities are reported, no information is available about the overall number of cases and deaths occurring among them. Consequently, the statistics on incidence and deaths due to diarrhoea diseases reported by the states and union territories are incomplete and unreliable. Further, the data reported under the subhead of cholera, dysentery, and gastroenteritis do not indicate the problem caused by other diarrhoea diseases.

Malaria was effectively controlled in the country by the mid 1960s under the National Malaria Control Programme. After its resurgence in the 1970s, a modified malaria control programmes was introduced in 1976. As indicated earlier, both the number of cases and the deaths due to malaria declined steeply in the country over the past 35 years. The incidence of malaria has, however, increased notably in Orissa, Gujarat and Tamil Nadu. Lack of adherence to scheduled spraying operations on scientific lines, management failures, biological resistance of vectors and parasites, and inadequate cleanliness are some of the underlying reasons for the resurgence of the diseases.

Acute respiratory infection (ARI) constitutes a complex and heterogeneous group of illnesses with the three conditions—bronchiolitis, acute laryngitis, and pneumonia—being primarily responsible for majority of ARI related deaths. In India, there was 33 lakh cases of ARI reported in 1983 as influenza, whooping cough, diptheria, and measles.

Tuberculosis continues to be a major health problem. Operations to control it were augmented considerably by ensuring the required quantities and quality of ante-TB drugs and equipment. Examination of sputum at the PHCs is being pursued with vigour on a target oriented basis. This is backed by a network of 358 district TB centres, 300 TB clinics, and 45000 TB beds in the country.

There are a number of other programmes to control and eradicate diseases like blindness, leprosy, fileria, Kala-azar etc. With increasing population pressure on the one hand, and constant degradation of environment on the other it has become necessary to improve surveillance of various diseases in the country, particularly in areas which are endemic to them.

MATERNAL AND CHILD HEALTH AND FAMILY WELFARE ASPECTS

One of the important aspects of the health care system is to safeguard the women from maternal mortality and the child. The maternal and child health care services are provided as a part of total health care to the community through the MCM centres and the existing health infrastructure in both rural and urban areas.

The medical attention received by mothers at the time of delivery is an important factor in controlling infant mortality and maternal mortality rates. The percentage of births attended by trained persons in rural India increased from 26.3% in 1981 to 30.5% in 19685, while in urban India the proportion increased from 65.8% to 72.3% during the same time span. Consequently, the infant mortality rate in rural areas declined from 138 in 1971 to 102 in 1988. The maternal mortality (deaths of women due to puerperal causes to total deaths) has, however, fluctuated around one per cent in the rural areas since 1981. Maternal under-nutrition, closely spaced pregnancies, severe anaemia, adolescent pregnancies, antenatal infections, and maternal hypertensions are some other factors which affects both the mother and the child during pregnancies.

HEALTH INFRASTRUCTURE

It was indicated earlier that the health care system from the curative viewpoint has greatly expanded in the country. Under the minimum needs programme, population norms were revised for the establishment of community health centres (CHCs) (a 30 bedded hospital with four basic specialities including a gynaecologist and a paediatrician), PHCs and subcentres. Under these norms there should be one sub-centre for every 5000 population, one PHC for every 30000 population, and one CHC for every 100000 population. There have, however, been several difficulties faced in the utilization of these services by the rural people and urban poor. For example, it has been founded in several surveys that 'services of PMCs have mostly been utilised by people living in a radius of about 5 km. Only people living at a distance from the PHC are hardly able to get the services when urgently needed. Although, provision has been made for the specialists at the CHC and at least three doctors (one of them to be a lady doctor) at each PHC, but a large number of posts remain vacant as people are not prepared to serve in villages, particularly in those that are located in tribal/hilly/or difficult areas. It is generally complained that most often the necessary drugs are not available in the PHCs and subcentres. The subcentres are usually manned by the ANM only, and, very often, she has to cover several villages. The appointment of multi-purpose health workers (one male and one female) in the subcentres should improve the current situation, but it is doubtful whether the type of training they receive is enough to prepare them suited to the job entrusted to them. One of the major issues with the health delivery system in the rural areas is that the masses have little confidence in the government health system. Those who can afford prefer to go to private doctors for treatment. The situation can be improved by developing an effective "health information System".

There are many other questions which need attention to ensure "Health for All" in the country. Time does not permit me to go into those issues. I shall now speak on strategies to attain health for all.

"STRATEGIES TO ATTAIN HEALTH FOR ALL BY 2000 AD"

After signing the Alma Ata declaration in 1978 at the International Conference on Primary Health Care, several steps were taken in the early eighties to achieve the above goal. Based on the recommendations of the Working Group on Health, the Sixth Five Year Plan adopted the following strategies:

(a) Emphasis to be shifted from development of city based curative services and super-specialities to tackling rural health problems.

A rural health care system based on a combination of preventive, promotive and curative health care system to be built up starting from the village as the base.

(b) The infrastructure for rural health care to consist of PHCs each serving a population of 30000 and subcentres each serving a population of 5000. These norms would be relaxed in hilly and tribal areas. The village or a population of 1000 would form the basic unit where there would be a trained health volunteer chosen by the community.

(c) Facilities for treatment in basic specialities to be provided at the CHCs at the block level for a population of one lakh with a 30 bedded hospital attached. A system of referral of cases from the CHC to the district hospital/medical college hospitals will be introduced.

(d) Various programmes under education, water supply and sanitation, control of communicable diseases, family planning maternal and child health care, nutrition and school health implemented by different departments/agencies would be properly coordinated for optimum results.

(e) Adequate medical and paramedical manpower to be trained for meeting the requirements of a programme of this order and all education and training programmes will be given suitable orientation towards rural health care.

(f) The people would be involved in tackling their health problems and community participation in the health programmes would be encouraged.

(g) The expanded immunization programme and the programme of prophylaxis against iron and vitamin A deficiencies would be strengthened. All the national public health schemes like malaria control, leprosy control, TB control, etc. would be monitored towards the specific goal adequate health care for all.

The Indian Council of Social Science Research and the Indian Council of Medical Research jointly constituted a "group" to bring the health practitioners and social scientists together to study the social aspects of medicine and suggest in alternative strategy to achieve Health for All. The Ministry of Health and Family Welfare devised a National Health Policy in 1983 covering various health and manpower developments aspects. The Seventh Five Year Plan further elaborated the objectives, goals and strategies for organising health care in the country. The Plan again emphasized that the Minimum Needs Programme would continue to be the sheet-anchor for the promotion of the primary health measures. Serious efforts for effective coordination and coupling of health and health related services and activities, e.g. nutrition, safe drinking water supply and sanitation, housing, education information and communication and social welfare will be made a part of the package for achieving the goal. Priority would be accorded to ensure active people's involvement, involvement of voluntary organisations and community participation in various health programmes besides the aspects of control of communicable and non-communicable diseases, medical education and medical and para-medical manpower etc.

The Government of India, Ministry of Health and Family Welfare, prepared a "pretesting Report" in May 1990 for second Evaluation of the "Strategies for Health for all by the Year 2000" as required by the World Health Organisation. According to this report there has been no alternations in the guiding principles; hence the plan of action for "Health for All" remains the same. It has, however, been decided to strengthen further certain identified areas. For example, in future, there will be consolidation of the rural health infrastructure which have already been created and the quality of services in them would be greatly improved. The urban health services will be further streamlined to avoid duplication of services and to extend the facilities to the people living in slum areas. To eliminate compartmentalisation in activities in respect of inter-sectorial and intra-sectorial coordination, mechanism has now been developed for strengthening such coordination in programme monitoring and evaluation. Mechanisms have also been developed for strengthening involvement of community/non-governmental organisations/voluntary organisations in planning, programmes implementation and evaluation of the National Health Programmes including primary health care delivery system.

Some of the obstacles impeding the speed of converted implementation relate to (i) constraints regarding finances; (ii) compartmentalisation in activities in respect of intersectoral and intra-sectorial coordination; (iii) inadequacy of information system and institution of timely corrective measures; and (iv) inadequate community participation in some areas.

It may be pointed out here that although safe drinking water and sanitation form priority programmes, as indicated earlier, we have largely paid lip services to the sanitation programmes, particularly in the rural areas. I consider it as a major factor which will continue to impede progress of health. This also becomes a basic issue from environmental viewpoint. Secondly, our data base on morbidity pattern has continued to remain very weak. We do not have complete information on age pattern of morbidity and the number of episodes of various diseases per person per annum. As many people do not go to formal systems of medical care every time, it is almost impossible to have a correct assessment of the situation in the country at any point of time.

Thirdly, there are certain areas which are endemic to particular diseases. Proper identification of those areas diseasewise and vigorous steps to control/eradicate the diseases from such areas are necessary.

Fourthly, it is necessary to evaluate and monitor properly the V.H.G. and M.P.W. Programme. It is learnt that many V.H.G. are now claiming themselves are medical practitioners having sanction of the central government. If a training of a few weeks can make people as medical practitioner and they start prescribing scheduled drugs (which cannot be given without doctors prescription) and dispensing all types of injections, a practice which must be stopped forthwith, what is the harm in having licentiates in medicine who would do much better job than these V.H.Gs. Similarly, a visit of a number of subcentres in May 1989 in Himachal Pradesh brought to light the weakness of the M.P.W. programme. A number of them do not have a male or female M.P.W. Moreover, their training of six months does not seem to be sufficient to prepare them for the job they are expected to perform. In some centres, the M.P.Ws did not have any idea as to what the U.N.I.C.E.F. kit contained.

Finally, as pointed out earlier, those who are able to afford do not seek medical help from the government run systems but prefer going to private medical practitioners. Many times the necessary drugs are not available at the government run dispensaries and hospitals. Many times doctors and paramedical persons are not available when there is emergency. There has to be increased community and voluntary agencies involvement on the one hand and building of confidence in the government-run system on the other.

3

THE GREEN REVOLUTION AND HEALTH

Dr. Fathima Kutty Kapil

I would like to depict about Green Revolution for good health because prevention of diseases is better than cure. The Green Revolution from rural areas can be brought back to the cities. The craze for garden and greenery can be created by 2,000 A.D. The atmosphere is polluted with industrial pollution in the cities. There is lack of fresh air and oxygen in the atmosphere due to industrial pollution. This can be eradicated to a great extent by growing plants and trees since the plants taken in carbide-oxide and leaves out oxygen.

Plants also give lots of joy and peace for a person who returns from heavy work. The peace and joy which is derived from the plants also in an indirect way gives good health.

In homes and balconies, in verandahs and gardens urban Indians can grow plants. The rooves of the houses can be beautified by growing creepers. These creepers catch the atmospheric dust which is the enemy of lungs and keep the fresh air to enter in. These plants prevent wind erosion.

The houses which have 10 yard can grow a few coconut plants and papaya. Papaya fruit give very good vitamins to health and fresh fruit from the plant have cent per cent of vitamins without getting perished. It is the only fruit which is permitted by the diabetes patients as part of their meal. A little kitchen garden can be grown which gives a lot of pleasure and recreation. Again the fresh vegetables from our garden not only provides timely needs but also we get the vitamins without perishing. The balconies can be decorated with creepers and plants. The little cemented places can be beautifully decorated with plants.

The growing green awareness can be created by seed suppliers, land scape, designers, pesticide suppliers, weed controllers, suppliers of garden equipment, coaching classes for bonsai etc.

Just 10 years ago the garden was the proverbial backyard of the house, but now it has become interior decoration. It can further be developed by growing plants in the portico. Nothing gives greater peace of mind than nature. The consciousness had to grow.

Nurseries have sprouted in urban areas. Plants are available to suit all pockets. A money plants or a fern is available for Rs. 15/-. The otherway of growing plants is interchanging and collection of plants from neighbours and friends. The nursing of plant can be spent as a recreation and hobby.

The plantation programmes are carried out throughout India but still many of the roads are without avenues. Though the Municipality take plantation programme, some of the roads go without plantation and out of the roads which have been planted a few survive and a few perish. So this plantation programme can be given incharge for each locality people.

These plants or avenues are essential not only for shade, fresh breeze, cooling and oxygen but it also prevents erosion which is created by the wind. It catches the atmospheric dust and provides fresh air and prevents nose and lung congestion.

In India Today (15th dated) it says "It was hardly surprising that greening in Bombay began in cuffe parade, a concrete jungle of high-rise apartments standing cheek-to-cheek like Californian giant redwoods shorn of foliage. Residents came together to develop an emerald patch called colaba woods, setting the trend for other private initiatives. Examples : Bandara's carter Road, Breach Candy and Napean Sea Road in Bombay."

Visakhapatnam also grows in apartments and multistoryed office buildings. The greenery in these apartments and multistoryed office buildings need to be developed by 2000 A.D. The greenery not only gives pleasantness to eyes but also cools the building.

Hence I conclude by saying Green Revolution provides Health for all and it can be improved by 2000 A.D. in Urban area.

4

HEALTH AS AN INDICATOR OF HUMAN RESOURCES DEVELOPMENT : A STUDY OF ANDHRA PRADESH

Prof. K.S. Chalam and D. Francis

Health is an important factor in the formation of human resources development which will play a vital role in improving the qualities of human beings who are the active agents of economic development. Improving the qualities of human agents contributes to labour productivity and to allocative and entrepreneurial ability[1]. Health measures also enhance the quality of human resources in addition to food and better shelter, especially in underdeveloped countries[2]. Therefore, any measure of development achievement in a nation must reflect the state of personal health in the nation.[3]

Ill-health causes a great loss of output and therefore any measure taken up to improve health rises the productivity of labour and also total output[4]. Improvement in health would promote learning, reduce absenteeism, improve stamina and increase energy output. Therefore, better health would contribute to improving the economic status of the poor and for expanding total output[5]. However, there is no agreed definition of health and there are no yardsticks for measuring it. It is a man's normal condition[6]. However, in its broader concept health has been emerging in many countries as that of improving the overall "quality of life" which has been defined as "condition of life resulting from the combination of the effects of the complete range of factors such as those determining health happiness (including comfort in the physical environment and a satisfying occupation), education, social and intellectual attainments, freedom of action, justice and freedom from oppression[7].

HEALTH POLICY

In recent decades the concept of health has become the most pressing issues of public policy. Most of the third World Countries are striving tor a better policy. And many a number of policy have been formulated before and after India attained Independence. In 1943, Health Survey and Development Committee known as Bhore Committee was appointed by the government of India to make a survey of the existing situation in regard to health conditions and health organisations prevailing in the country. Some of its recommendations are (i) health services should provide consultant, laboratory and institutional facilities for proper diagnosis and treatment, (ii) health programme should lay emphasis on preventive work.

Since the Bhore Committee report, there has been a tremendous change in the problems connected with health administrations[5]. Now it has been well recognized that in terms of resources for economic development nothing can be considered of higher importance thus the health of the people.

A concrete shape to the health policy was later given with the setting up of Planning Commission in 1950 as a part of the overall social and economic development of the country. The Committee 'Health Survey and Planning Committee' popularly known as Mudaliar Committee appointed by the government of India in 1961 made some recommendations for future planning of health development in India. It recommended that there should be one doctor for every 3500 population (1:3500) and the ideal bed population ratio according to the committee was 1:1000. It also touched upon other items like nurses, pharmacists and other personnel".

The constitution of India aims at the elimination of poverty, ignorance and ill-health and directs the state with regard to the raising of the level of nutrition and the standard of its people and the improvement of public health as among its primary duties. It is also stated that securing the health and strength of workers, men and women, specially ensuring that children are given opportunities and facilities to develop.

A National Health Policy[10] was formulated in 1983 after examining the existing situation of health in the country and with a view to attain the committed goal of "Health for all by the year 2000

A.D." through the Universal provision of comprehensive primary health care services. It has identified the need for providing primary health care with special emphasis on the preventive, promotive and rehabilitative aspects. It seeks to provide universal, comprehensive primary health care services, relevant to the actual needs and priorities of the community. Also it attributes higher priority to the promotion of family planning as people's programme on a voluntary basis. The Programme also places high emphasis on the supply of drinking water to all problem villages, improvements in the housing and environments of the weaker sections of society, spread of elementary education, etc.

METHODOLOGY

To construct human resources development of health the different systems of medicine considered in the study are Allopathic, Ayurveda, Unani, and Homeopathy. The Physical facilities examined in the study are, hospitals and dispensaries, beds in the hospitals and doctors. Therefore doctors existing under different systems of medicine are combined and converted into hospital beds which is considered as a single unit of health services index i.e. weighted index of health (WIH).

The criteria for conversion of doctors into beds were obtained from government reports of the medical and health department. The number of doctors existing in each district is multiplied with their bed-doctor ratios for the years 1961, 1971 and 1981 respectively. The hospital beds so obtained are combined with the already existing number of hospital beds which gives the total number of hospital beds for each district, the resultant index in terms of hospital beds has been expressed per 10000 population.

i.e. WIH = B + WD

Where B = Beds

W = Weights

D = Doctors

The Human Resources Development Index of Health and its Variations in the Districts of Andhra Pradesh

A weighted index of health (WIH) has been constructed to study the physical facilities of health which constitute a past of human resources development and also to find out the gap between the districts in the formation of physical health facilities in Andhra Pradesh.

The index shows that there are considerable variations in the formation of health facilities in the districts of the state in 1961, 1971 and also in 1981. The data are presented in Table 1. In 1961, Hyderabad district tops the position with 232.08 index. It is found that the index of Hyderabad district is four times higher than the State average. The lowest position in the index is shown by Nalgonda district with 17.02 which is far below the state average. These two districts are in Telangana region. The second position in the formation of physical health facilities is occupied by Visakhapatnam with 112.82 followed by Kurnool with 103.25 and Guntur with 71.38. This may be due to the fact that there exist teaching hospitals in these districts. Therefore, the index is found to be higher. The teaching hospitals in these districts may be rendering better services for improvement in the health of the people.

There is only one district, Chittoor whose performance in the formation of human resources development is found to be above the state average (60.51) without a teaching hospital. Therefore, the number of districts which are above the state average out of 20 comes to five. The index for Nellore is also nearly equal to the state average. The remaining 14 districts appear poor in the formatting of health facilities in their respective districts when compared with the state average during 1961.

The human resources development index in the regions of the state shows that there are two regions out of four whose average index is less than the state average. They are Coastal Andhra and Telangana.

The above mentioned five districts are also found to be above the state average in 1961 even in terms of districts mean. The variation between the districts is more than 90% (C.V.=93.26). This shows that each district in the state is varying 93% from the state average index of human resources development in health.

The performance of the districts in the formation of health facilities in most of the districts have not been improved during 1961 and 1971. The index has declined during this period. This can be observed from the variations in the weighted index of health presented in Table 2. However, the highest position continues to be enjoyed by

Hyderabad whose performance is three times more than that of the state's average. But the lowest position in the index has not remained the same as in the previous period 1961. The position has shifted to Mahbubnagar which also falls in Telangana region. The index of this district is 6.4 times less than that of Hyderabad. There are six districts, viz. Visakhapatnam, Guntur, Nellore, Kurnool, Chittoor and Warangal whose indices of health are above the human resources development index of the state. The existence of teaching hospitals at the head quarters of Warangal during this period brought Warangal to the above state average status in 1971. Though, there is no teaching hospital in Nellore district, the performance in the formation of health facilities is much improved when compared to the state average in 1971. The change in the position of the index may indicate an improvement in the physical facilities of health.

It is worth noting that there are only six districts who have improved their performance during the period 1961-1971. They are Medak, Mahaboobnagar, Nalgonda, Warangal, Khammam and Adilabad. All these districts are in Telangana region. The remaining 178 districts did not show any improvement during the period. The region wise analysis shows that there is only one region, Telangana whose index is above the state average.

It is also found that the index of human resources has declined in some districts during 1961-1971. They are Visakhapatnam with 1.5 times and 1.2 times each in Kurnool and Hyderabad. Further, there is a reduction in the coefficient of variation by 36% in the districts. The variation has been narrowed down during 1961-1971, i.e the formation in the physical facilities of health have been improving evenly in the districts during the period.

The physical facilities created during the year 1981 has not been improved in the districts when compared to 1961 and 1971. The indices are still declining. There is a sudden fall in the human resources development index of health in all the districts in 1981. The top position of Hyderabad district is unaltered, but it is interesting to see that the lowest position has shifted from Telangana region to Coastal Andhra. Prakasam in Coastal Andhra has this value now. The seven districts which continue to be above the state average are the same, Hyderabad, Visakhapatnam, Kurnool, Guntur, Nellore, Chittoor and Warangal. There is only one district East Godavari which is just above the state average. Its index is 16.68. It has improved its relative position in 1981 though the physical index has declined during 1961-1981.

The region wise indices indicate that the position has remained the same. However, East Godavari district has joined the above state average districts in 1981. The remaining 13 districts continue to fall below the average of the state and district mean.

Thus the study show that though there is no improvement in the formation of physical facilities in all the districts during 1961-1981. Telangana region is found to be more effective in the formation of health facilities than that of the other regions.

The coefficient of variation and standard deviation computed for the period 1961, 1971 and 1981 indicate that there is no uniform decline or increase in the even distribution of health facilities among the districts in the state. This may be due to lack of a perspective plan in the development of health facilities in the districts. This is also due to the 'adhocism' of the government dealing with the health status of the people in Andhra Pradesh.

CONCLUSION

Health plays a vital role for improvement in the quality of life. The facilities created in an area are responsible for the health of the people. To study the health facilities created in the state, we have estimated an index: human resources development index of health.

The human resources development index of health shows a declining trend in the formation of health facilities over the period. The growth of the index over the period is found to be negative. This may be due to increase in the number of people and also the bed-patient norms set by the government. Hyderabad district tops the list of human resources development index of health for the three periods studied here. But the lowest position has not been found to be occupied by the same district over the period. The Telengana region is found to be better placed in the formation of human resources development of health in terms of the magnitude and growth of the human resources development indices of districts. Though, the inequalities among the districts have come down over the periods, the coefficient of variation (C.V.) and Standard Deviation (S.D.) shows that there is no uniform decline or increase in the even distribution of health facilities among the districts in the state. This is due to the 'adhocism' of the government in dealing with the health status of the people in Andhra Pradesh.

REFERENCES

1. Schub, G.E.. et al., "Food Aid and Human Capital Formation", *Food and Development,* Agricultural Development Council, INC, New York, 1981, p. 51.
2. Schultz, T.w. "Investment in Human Capital", *American Economic Review,* Vol. 51, No. 1, 1961, pp. 1-17.
3. Malenbaum, W., "Health and Productivity in Poor Areas", *Empirical Studies in Health Economics,* Klarman, H.E., (Ed), John Hopkins University Press, London, 1974, pp. 31-33.
4. Panchamukhi, P.R., "Economics of Health" : A Trend Report, A Survey of Research in Economics, Vol. VI, Infrastructure, ICSSR, Allied, New Delhi, 1980, p. 247.
5. Golladay, F., *Health Problems and Policies in Developing Countries,* Staff working paper No. 412, World Bank, Aug. 1980.
6. Park, J.E. & Park, K., Text Book of Preventive and Social Medicine Bansari Das Bhanot, Jabalpur, 1979, p.12.
7. WHO, "Health Aspects of Human Settlements", *Public Health papers* No. 66, 1977.
8. Government of India, *The Gazetteer of India Vol. IV, Administration and Public Welfare,* Ministry of Education and Social Welfare, New Delhi, 1978, p. 584-5.
9. Govt. of Andhra Pradesh, *Sixth Five Year Plan 1980-85 Andhra Pradesh,* Draft Vol. II, Finance & Planning Dept., Hyderabad, p. 346.
10. Government of India, *National Health Policy,* Appendix VI, Ministry Health and Family Welfare, 1983, pp. 33-49.

Table 1 : Weighted Index of Health (WIH)

District	1961	1971	1981
1	2	3	4
1. Srikakulam	25.79	20.07	9.87
2. Vizianagaram	-	-	9.07
3. Visakhapatnam	112.82	46.41	23.35
North Coastal Andhra	68.83	33.78	15.13
4. East Godavari	42.26	33.31	16.68
5. West Godavari	36.58	25.86	10.06
6. Krishna	47.39	34.09	15.66
7. Guntur	71.38	48.47	19.15
8. Prakasam	-	24.40	8.97
9. Nellore	55.54	46.51	17.19
Coastal Andhra	52.00	35.71	14.92
10. Kurnool	103.25	53.02	20.99
11. Anantarpur	86.34	25.61	11.14
12. Cuddapah	37.10	31.83	12.89
13. Chittoor	60.59	37.43	15.66
Rayalaseema			
14. Hyderabad	232.08	116.03	78.52
15. Ranga Reddy	-	-	11.83
16. Nizamabad	27.02	24.03	11.09
17. Medak	18.50	23.68	10.81
18. Mehaboobnagar	19.94	18.05	9.85
19. Nalgonda	17.02	23.09	11.00
20. Warangal	30.26	43.59	20.80
21. Khammam	23.65	26.04	10.55
22. Karimnagar	18.96	18.72	9.85
23. Adilabad	29.68	33.77	13.95
Telangana	56.61	42.04	19.66
Andhra Pradesh	57.64	38.09	16.86
Number of districts	20	21	23
Mean ($\bar{X}$)	52.30	36.03	16.54
Standard Deviation (σ)	48.78	20.66	13.87
Coefficient of variation (CV)	93.26	57.36	83.85

Table 2 : Percentage change in the Human Resources Development Weighted Index of Health (WIH)

	District	*1961-71*	*1971-81*	*1961-81*
	1	*2*	*3*	*4*
1.	Srikakulam	-28.50	-103.34	-161.30
2.	Vizianagaram	-	-	-
3.	Visakhapatanam	-143.09	-98.76	-383.17
	North Coastal Andhra	-103.76	-123.26	-354.17
4.	East Godavari	-26.87	-99.70	-153.36
5.	West Godavari	-41.45	-157.06	-263.62
6.	Krishna	-39.01	-117.69	-202.62
7.	Guntur	-44.29	-158.33	-272.74
8.	Prakasam	-	-172.02	-
9.	Nellore	-19.41	-170.56	-223.09
	Coastal Andhra	-45.62	-139.34	-248.52
10.	Kurnool	-94.74	-152.60	-391.90
11.	Anantapur	-41.90	-129.89	-226.21
12.	Cuddapah	-18.23	-146.94	-187.32
13.	Chittoor	-56.11	-126.27	-253.24
	Rayalaseema	-64.55	-139.02	-239.29
14.	Hyderabad	-100.02	-47.77	-195.57
15.	Ranga Reddy	-	-	-
16.	Nizamabad	-11.19	-119.11	-142.64
17.	Medak	28.00*	-119.06	-71.14
18.	Mahaboobnagar	10.47*	-83.25	-102.44
19.	Nalgonda	35.68*	-109.91	-54.73
20.	Warangal	444.05*	-109.57	-45.48
21.	Khammam	10.10*	-146.82	-124.17
22.	Karimnagar	-1.28	-90.05	-92.49
23.	Adilabad	13.78*	-142.08	-112.76
Tenangana		-34.66	-113.83	-187.95
Andhra Pradesh		-51.33	-125.92	-241.87

*Percentage change is positive

SECTION B

DEMOGRAPHIC ASPECTS OF HEALTH PLANNING

5

INTER-DISTRICT VARIATIONS IN HEALTH SERVICES IN ANDHRA PRADESH

Prof. G. Ramachandrudu and Dr. G. Venkata Rao

INTRODUCTION

Since Independence, the Government are providing the medical facilities which directly curbed the spread of communicable diseases like plague, cholera, typohoid, etc. Eventhough significant strides in health care took place the Government couldn't eradicate the diseases like typhoid, malaria, small pox, etc., because of insufficient, infrastructure facilities especially in rural areas. It indirectly lead to child mortality, thereby increased the fertility rate to substitute the children lost, then it leads to higher growth rate of population which is an obstacle to socio-economic development. The acceptance of Family Planning methods depends on number of factors, especially the medical aid provide by the Government before and after sterilisation. If the facilities are more, generally, the family planning acceptance will be more. This paper analyses the inter-district variation in the Health infrastructure facilities which are available in A.P. at three point of times, i.e., 1965, 75 and 85. The paper also examines the relationship between health infrastructure and couple protection rate with the inter-district cross-section data. The data used in this study are secondary data taken from Statistical Abstracts of Andhra Pradesh and Health Statistics of Andhra Pradesh Published by Government of Andhra Pradesh.

GROWTH OF THE SUPPLY OF HEALTH SERVICES IN ANDHRA PRADESH

We can observe for the table 1, that as there is an all time growth of almost all the health services, there is 14.19 per cent decline in the number of beds available during 1965-75. The highest growth is recorded in the number of doctors during 1975-85, the percentage growth being 47.84.

There is 26.16% growth in the number of hospitals and dispensaries during 1965-75, and it is 6.06 during 1975-85.

There is a 14.19% decline in the number of beds available during 1965-75, whereas there is a 25.42% growth during 1975-85.

There is a 12.65% growth in the number of doctors during 1965-75, and there is a record growth of 47.84% during 1975-85.

Table 1 : Number of Hospitals and Dispensaries, number of beds available and number of doctors in Andhra Pradesh in three different periods

Year	*No. of Hospitals and Dispensaries*	*%*	*No. of Beds available*	*%*	*No. of Doctors*	*%*
1965	1124	-	25682	-	3305	-
1975	1418	26.16	22039	-14.19	3723	12.65
1985	1504	6.06	27642	+25.42	5504	47.84

Source : Statistical Abstracts of Andhra Pradesh, 1965, 75, 85.

In order to analyse the inter-district variation in health inputs utilised the statistical methods like Arithmetic mean, standard deviation and coefficient of variation.

INTER-DISTRICT VARIATION IN THE NUMBER OF HOSPITALS AND DISPENSARIES IN ANDHRA PRADESH

The expansion of health sector can be measured by both the establishment of a dispensary and improving the infrastructure of it. Thus the primary responsibility of the Government is to open new hospitals and dispensaries in rural areas of the State.

Table 2 presents the comparison of Hospitals and Dispensaries in three point of times, i.e., 1965, 1975 and 1985 in Andhra Pradesh. In 1965, the State capital Hyderabad occupied first place with 117 Hospitals and Dispensaries. The second place occupied by Kurnool with 103 hospitals and dispensaries. East Godavari District in the third place with 98 hospitals and dispensaries. Khammam is in the last place with 22 hospitals and dispensaries. Thc total no. of hospitals and dispensaries in the State is 1124. In the year 1975, East Godavari district occupied first place with 127 hospitals and dispensaries. The second place goes to Visakhapatnam district with 126 hospitals and dispensaries. The third place is occupied by the district Nellore with 114 hospitals and dispensaries. In 1985, East Godavari District still continue its first place with 131 hospitals and dispensaries. The Nellore district comes second place with 127 hospitals and dispensaries. The third place goes to Cuddapah district with 114 hospitals and dispensaries.

Thus we observed that there are wide variations among the districts in health infrastructural facilities like hospitals and dispensaries in Andhra Pradesh.

INTER-DISTRICT VARIATIONS IN THE NUMBER OF BEDS AVAILABLE

Table 3 presents the availability of beds position in various hospitals and dispensaries. Visakhapatnam district is in second position in 1965 with 3459 beds available in various hospitals and dispensaries. The first place is occupied by Hyderabad with 4797 beds available in hospitals and dispensaries. Guntur district is in third place with 2424 beds available. The availability of beds position changed in 1975. The city of Hyderabad still hold the first position with 5596 beds and the second and the third place goes to Visakhapatnam and Guntur districts with 2300 and 1493 beds available in various hospitals and dispensaries. In the year 1985, Hyderabad city still holds it continuity as first place in case of availability of beds which is 6232. Visakhapatnam district is in second place with 2414 beds and East Godavari district is in third place with 1704 beds.

The table reflects that the availability of beds is more in the districts in which there exists teaching hospitals. Correct picture may be evolved by deleting the beds in the teaching hospitals.

INTER-DISTRICT VARIATIONS IN THE NUMBER OF DOCTORS AVAILABLE

Table 4 reveals the availability of Number of Doctors in the districts in three different times, namely, 1965, 1975 and 1985. Hyderabad city is ahead of all the districts in case of doctors in 1965.

The second place is occupied by Visakhapatnam with 441 doctors. Third place goes to Kurnool with 312 doctors. In 1975, Hyderabad is in first place with 838 doctors. The second place goes to Visakhapatnam district with 347 doctors and third place occupied by Guntur district with 326 doctors. In 1985 the first, second and third places occupied by Hyderabad, East Godavari and Guntur districts with 1068, 469 and 434 doctors.

Thus again the districts with teaching hospitals dominate the scene of the availability of doctors. If we add private medical practitioners, urban districts would definitely lead the availability of doctors.

INTER-DISTRICT VARIATIONS IN DOCTORS-BED RATIO

Table 5 presents the doctor-bed ratio in three different periods i.e., 1965, 1975 and 1985. In 1965 Nizamabad district is the highest doctor-bed ratio of 1:17.4. The second place occupied by Cuddapah district with 1:17.16 doctors bed ratio. The third place occupied by West Godavari district with 1:15.9. In 1975 and 1985, the doctor bed ratio is slightly improved. In 1975 Nellore district is in the highest position with 1:8.47. The second place goes to Anantapur district with 1:8.44. Krishna district is in the third place with 1:7.44. In 1985, the doctor-bed ratio is highest in Ranga Reddy district with 1:7.39. The second place by Krishna district with 1:7.17 and third place by Anantapur district with 1:6.26.

Thus we have observed that the variation in the doctor-bed ratio is not similar to that the earlier measures of health facilities.

INTER-DISTRICT VARIATIONS IN HOSPITAL-DOCTOR RATIO

Table 6 presents the Doctor Hospital Ratios in the districts of Andhra Pradesh in three point of times, i.e., 1965, 1975 and 1985. Hyderabad district has the highest hospital doctor ratio i.e., 1:7.6 in 1965. The second place occupied by the Guntur district 1:4.93 hospital doctor ratio. The third place goes to Visakhapatnam district with 1:4.64. In 1975, the doctor hospital ratio has increased in Hyderabad city from 1:7.6 to 1:11.32 and further increased to 1:13.19 in 1985. The second place is occupied by the Warangal district with 1:6.02 in 1975 and increased to 1:7.18 in 1985 which occupied the same position as in 1975. The third place goes to Guntur district with 1:15.53 hospital doctor ratio. It is increased to 1:6.48 in 1985, occupied the same position as in 1975.

MEASURES OF DISPERSION OF HEALTH SERVICES IN A.P.

Table 7 presents mean, S.D. and C.V. of health services in Andhra Pradesh in the years 1965, 1975 and 1985. Altogether four variables representing different indices of health services are presented in the table. The variables are :

1. Hospitals and dispensaries in Andhra Pradesh
2. Number of beds available in all hospitals and dispensaries.
3. Number of doctors available.
4. Doctors, Medical Dispensaries and Hospitals.

An interesting feature of health services in Andhra Pradesh is that the average number of hospitals and dispensaries have declined from 67.5 in 1975 to 65.39 in 1985. Similarly the average number of beds available has declined from 1284.1 in 1965 to 1201.3 in 1985. However, average number of doctors has continuously increased from 165.25 in 1965 to 177.29 in 1975 to 239.30 in 1985.

Standard Deviation and C.V. indicate the inter-district variations and changes thereof during 1965 to 1985. With regard to hospital beds and dispensaries S.D. has increased from 5.9 in 1965 to 9.29 in 1975 to 8.95 in 1985. Similarly the C.V. also has increased from 10.49 in 1965 to 13.75 in 1975 to 13.69 in 1985.

In case of number of beds available, the average number of beds available has decline from 1284.1 in 1965 to 1049.47 in 1975 and again increased to 1201.83 in 1985. The standard deviation and coefficient of variation in case of beds availability has also maintained the same tendency as average beds available in various hospitals, and dispensaries. The standard deviation, which declined from 343.27 in 1965 to 244.39 in 1975 and slightly increased to 246.10 in 1985. The coefficient of variation in regard to beds availability, it continuously declined, from 26.73 in 1965 to 23.29 in 1975 and 20.48 in 1985.

In the case of number of doctors available, the average number of doctors increased from 165.25 in 1965 to 177.29 in 1975 to 239.30 in 1985. The standard deviation of number of doctors also declined from 44.25 in 1965 to 34.00 in 1975 and increased to 43.94 in 1985. The coefficient of variation of number of doctors available continuously declined from 26.78 in 1965 to 19.17 in 1975 and to 18.36 in 1985.

The average number of doctors, medical dispensaries and hospitals are 239.30 in 1985. The standard deviation of these variables are 43.94 and the coefficient of variation in 1836.

Thus, we may conclude that inter-district variations with regard to the hospitals and dispensaries is increasing whereas the variations in the number of beds available and the number of doctors is decreasing.

CORRELATION BETWEEN THE COUPLE PROTECTION RATES AND THE HEALTH SERVICES

Table 8 presents zero order correlation coefficient between the couple protection rate and the health inputs (infrastructural of health services). We can observe from the table that correlation between C.P.R. and hospital beds is the highest (0.63).

Next comes the correlation between dispensaries and C.P. Rate (0.45). Lastly, the correlation coefficient between doctors and couple protection rate is 0.43.

Thus, we may conclude that there is an urgent need to reduce the disparities between the districts with regard to the availability of hospital beds which is highly correlated to the couple protection rate. Therefore, the success of family welfare programme depends on the availability and proper maintenance of health facilities together with the required staff for post-operative care.

Table 2 : Number of Hospitals and Dispensaries in Andhra Pradesh

(District-wise)

District	*Year*		
	1965	*1975*	*1985*
Srikakulam	77	75	59
Vizianagaram	-	-	60
Visakhapatnam	95	126	109
East Godavari	98	127	131
West Godavari	66	97	105
Krishna	50	46	52
Guntur	62	59	67
Prakasam	-	52	57
Nellore	62	114	127
Kurnool	103	77	83
Anantpur	45	50	58
Cuddapah	37	111	114
Chittoor	59	54	63
Ranga Reddy	-	-	27
Hyderabad	117	74	81
Nizamabad	33	32	26
Medak	25	55	34
Mehaboobnagar	40	48	48
Nalgonda	28	74	30
Warangal	39	35	40
Khammam	22	38	45
Karimnagar	29	42	43
Adilabad	37	32	45
Andhra Pradesh	1124	1418	1504

Source : Statistical Abstracts of A.P., 1965, 1975, 1985

Table 3 : Number of Beds Available in the District of Andhra Pradesh

(District-wise)

District	*Year*		
	1965	*1975*	*1985*
Srikakulam	311	498	663
Vizianagaram	-	-	365
Visakhapatnam	3459	2300	2414
East Godavari	2005	1303	1704
West Godavari	1127	638	762
Krishna	1031	937	1363
Guntur	2424	1493	1771
Prakasam	-	305	484
Nellore	1396	864	1039
Kurnool	1395	1199	1353
Anantpur	778	819	933
Cuddapah	824	538	681
Chittoor	1531	1216	1428
Ranga Reddy	-	-	658
Hyderabad	4797	5596	6232
Nizamabad	714	514	648
Medak	336	343	532
Mehaboobnagar	655	513	720
Nalgonda	572	603	653
Warangal	951	1102	1292
Khammam	706	388	569
Karimnagar	322	434	646
Adilabad	348	436	732
Andhra Pradesh	25682	22039	27642

Source : Statistical Abstracts of A.P., 1965, 1975, 1985

Table 4 : Number of Doctors available in the districts of Andhra Pradesh

(District-wise)

District	*Year*		
	1965	*1975*	*1985*
Srikakulam	89	94	115
Vizianagaram	-	-	129
Visakhapatnam	441	347	391
East Godavari	203	252	469
West Godavari	71	113	163
Krishna	77	126	190
Guntur	306	326	434
Prakasam	-	58	101
Nellore	96	102	168
Kurnool	312	260	358
Anantpur	75	97	149
Cuddapah	48	75	118
Chittoor	202	223	363
Ranga Reddy	-	-	89
Hyderabad	891	838	1068
Nizamabad	41	81	120
Medak	48	70	123
Mehaboobnagar	56	107	142
Nalgonda	43	85	140
Warangal	151	211	287
Khammam	48	84	118
Karimnagar	48	94	137
Adilabad	58	80	132
Andhra Pradesh	3305	3723	5504

Source : Statistical Abstracts of A.P., 1965, 1975, 1985

Table 5 : Inter-District Variations in Doctor-Bed Ratio in Andhra Pradesh

(District-wise)

District	*Year*		
	1965	*1975*	*1985*
Srikakulam	1:3.5	1:5.30	1:5.76
Vizianagaram	-	-	1:2.8
Visakhapatnam	1:7.8	1:6.2	1:6.17
East Godavari	1:9.8	1:5.17	1:3.63
West Godavari	1:15.9	1:5.64	1:4.67
Krishna	1:13.4	1:7.44	1:7.17
Guntur	1:7.9	1:4.58	1:4.08
Prakasam	-	1:5.26	1:4.79
Nellore	1:14.54	1:8.47	1:6.18
Kurnool	1:4.47	1:4.61	1:3.77
Anantpur	1:10.37	1:8.44	1:6.26
Cuddapah	1:17.16	1:7.13	1:5.77
Chittoor	1:7.57	1:5.45	1:3.93
Ranga Reddy	-	-	1:7.39
Hyderabad	1:5.4	1:6.68	1:5.84
Nizamabad	1:17.4	1:6.35	1:5.4
Medak	1:27.0	1:4.90	1:4.32
Mehaboobnagar	1:11.6	1:4.79	1:5.07
Nalgonda	1:13.30	1:7.10	1:4.66
Warangal	1:6.30	1:5.22	1:4.50
Khammam	1:14.70	1:4.61	1:4.82
Karimnagar	1:6.70	1:4.61	1:4.71
Adilabad	1:6.70	1:5.45	1:5.54
Andhra Pradesh	1:7.7	1:5.92	1:5.0

Source : Statistical Abstracts of A.P., 1965, 1975, 1985

Table 6 : Inter-District Variations in Hospital Doctor-Bed Ratio in Andhra Pradesh

(District-wise)

District	*Year*		
	1965	*1975*	*1985*
Srikakulam	1:1.50	1:1.25	1:1.95
Vizianagaram	-	-	1:2.15
Visakhapatnam	1:4.64	1:2.75	1:3.59
East Godavari	1:2.07	1:1.98	1:3.58
West Godavari	1:1.08	1:1.16	1:1.55
Krishna	1:1.54	1:2.74	1:3.65
Guntur	1:4.93	1:5.53	1:6.48
Prakasam	-	1:1.12	1:1.77
Nellore	1:1.55	1:0.89	1:1.32
Kurnool	1:3.02	1:3.38	1:4.31
Anantpur	1:1.66	1:1.94	1:2.57
Cuddapah	1:1.29	1:0.68	1:1.03
Chittoor	1:3.42	1:4.12	1:5.76
Ranga Reddy	-	-	1:3.30
Hyderabad	1:7.60	1:11.32	1:13.19
Nizamabad	1:1.24	1:2.53	1:4.62
Medak	1:1.92	1:1.27	1:3.62
Mehaboobnagar	1:1.40	1:2.23	1:2.96
Nalgonda	1:1.53	1:1.15	1:4.67
Warangal	1:3.87	1:6.02	1:7.18
Khammam	1:2.15	1:2.21	1:2.62
Karimnagar	1:1.66	1:2.24	1:3.19
Adilabad	1:1.57	1:2.50	1:2.93
Andhra Pradesh	1:1.30	1:2.63	1:3.66

Source : Statistical Abstracts of A.P., 1965, 1975, 1985

Table 7 : Mean, Standard Deviation and Coefficient of Variation of Health Services in Andhra Pradesh, 1965, 1975 and 1985

Item	*Year*	*Arithmetic Mean*	*Standard Deviation*	*Coefficient Variation*
1. Hospitals and Dispensaries	1965	56.2	5.9	10.49
	1975	67.52	9.29	13.75
	1985	65.39	8.95	13.69
2. Number of Beds available	1965	1284.1	343.27	26.73
	1975	1049.47	244.39	23.29
	1985	1201.83	246.10	20.48
3. Number of Doctors (Allopathic)	1965	165.25	44.5	26.78
	1975	177.29	34.00	19.17
	1985	239.30	43.94	18.36

Table 8 : Zero Order Correlation Coeffiicients between Couple Protection Rate and Health Inputs

Sl. No.	*Health Input*	*Correlation Coefficient*
1.	Numbers of Doctors	+0.43
2.	Numbers of Hospitals Beds	+ 0.63*
3.	Numbers of Dispensaries	+ 0.45

* Significant at 5% level.

6

DEMOGRAPHIC IMPLICATIONS OF HEALTH FOR ALL BY 2000 AD

Prof. PVS Sarma

India's population increased by 24.8% between the 1961 and 1971 censuses and 25% between the 1971 and 1981 censuses. It has been estimated that the population of India, which was 685.2 million in 1981, would increase to 837.2 million in 1991 and to 996.0 million in 2001. One redeeming feature is that the decade growth rate has more or less reached a plateau and is actually showing signs of a decline. As a consequences the annual growth rate will decline to 2% during (the period) 1981-1991 and to 1.6% during 1991-2001. The annual additions to the population are likely to be on the order of 15.24 million, 15.2 million and 14.57 million during the period 1986-1991, 1991-1996 and 1996-2001 respectively. Life expectancy at birth for 1980 has been estimated at 54.3 years for males and 54.7 years for females. It is expected that this will increase to 64.1 years for males and 65.6 years for females by the year 2001. The implications of the current growth rate of population in India for the overall socio-economic development of the country are well recognised. Steps, are, therefore, being taken to bring about a rapid decline in the birth rate.

The level of infant Mortality is widely used not only as a demographic measure, but also as an important indicator of the level of health in a society and indeed of its living standards in general. There are five demographic variables which have a substantial impact on the chances of survival of Infants and Young Children the age of the mother at the time of Birth, the child's sex and birth order, the inter-birth interval, and whether the birth was single or multiple. It is commonly accepted that males have higher mortality than females at all ages, except where maternal mortality is important.

Family Planning, including health care and welfare of mothers and children, has been acknowledged as a catalyst in and corollary to socio-economic developmental efforts. The national health policy provides the necessary direction for re-orienting and restructuring the health services with long term perspectives. The policy envisages a conceptual change from the emphasis on curative services to the preventive and promotive aspects of health care, particularly of the weaker and deprived sections of society. While envisaging health and human development as a vital component of overall integrated socio-economic development, the policy emphasises the need for ensuring adequate nutrition, safe drinking water and improved sanitation. The existing development planning model for India takes into account the interdependence between the pattern of population change and the pattern of development. India is committed to the goal of NRR (Net Reproduction Rate) of 1 by the year 2000. The performance under the programme during the Sixth Five Year Plan (1980-85) gives rise to the hope that, with the Government's firm commitment to and support of the programme on a priority basis, this goal will be realisable if the present momentum of the programme is maintained. The overall increase in the couple protection rate during this period was 45% or 10% points. Currently 40 million couples out of 126 million couples in the reproductive age group are effectively protected by (using) contraceptives.

With regard to different family planning methods, the performance of the country as a while during this period was around 80%. On the basis of the demographic goal of an NRR of 1 by the year 2000 targets have been laid down for the Seventh Five-Year Plan period (1985-1990), in terms of the couple protection rate, crude birth rate, crude death rate, annual growth rate, life expectancy a birth and infant mortality rate and also in terms of the level of performance which will be required regarding the different family planning methods such as sterilisation and conventional contraceptive, and for different programme activities under the MCH Programmes.

Family Planning Programmes have clearly lowered fertility in a number of developing countries. Fertility has declined most in countries where strong family planning programmes operate with Government support in favourable social and economic settings. When national family planning programme were not only to improve family health but also to reduce high rates of population growth that slow economic development.

Public health technology applied on a mass scale in the developing countries has reduced death rates dramatically. Government health expenditure in most developing countries are between 0.3 and 2.5% of GNP. The age and geographical distribution of the population also affects the health services. In a high-fertility community the primary stress on health services will be the care of mothers and children. The problems of medical treatment for infants are substantially greater than the problems of treating young adults. In a high-fertility region many woman have several pregnancies very early in their child bearing years and continue to bear children upto the time of menopause. Very young mothers, older mothers, mothers with closely spaced pregnancies all higher parity mothers-face risks.

Since 1950, food production in India has almost tripled, with the greatest increases occurring in the late sixties, after new high yielding seed varieties were introduced. But parallel with a phenomenal increase in food production, India's population has more than doubles. Although India has had a national family planning programme for more national family planning programmes for more than 30 years, only a few states have made real progress in reducing birth rates.

Even in areas like the Punjab, malnutrition did not disappear. Partly this was due to changes in land tenure which, combined with population pressures, squeezed poorer families off the land. Malnutrition remained worst among women and female children, a result of discriminatory patterns of food distribution within the family which are found throughout India.

In 1986, an estimated 45% of India's people suffered from some level of malnutrition. Much of current malnutrition is the result of the inability of large number of very poor families to buy food at market prices and the maldistribution of food within families. This situation is unlikely to improve very much unless broad-based rural and urban development, aided by further increases in agricultural and Industrial productivity, out paces future population growth.

"The quality of human life is inseparable from the quality of the environment. It is increasingly clear that both are inseparable from the question of human members and concentrations. One of the clearest lessons of the last two decades of work in population is that investments in women's status, access to eduction, health and the means of family planning not only improve the quality of life but the also the best and quickest way to reduce the population growth rates", says the population report.

According to UNFPA report, world population, currently 5.3 billion, will increase by another billion people during the 1990s. During the next century. It will probably double and could triple. The biggest increase will be in the poorest countries. Consequence for the environment and for development prospects will be serious; they could even be catastrophic.

The developing countries are doing their best to increase their share of industrial production and consumption. Thus their share of industrial pollution is rising, and will continue to rise. Developed or developing, the more people the more pollution, at any level of development, larger number consume more resources and produce more waste.

The report suggests the following action plans :

1. a shift to cleaner technologies, energy efficiency and resource conservation by all countries.
2. a direct and all out attack on poverty itself.
3. reducing population growth, especially in the countries with the highest rates of growth.

7

DEMOGRAPHIC ASPECTS OF RURAL HEALTH POLICY IN INDIA

Dr. G. Rama Rao

Organised and planned rural health care activities are vital for obviating the ill effects of major historical, political and socio-economic changes. This is particularly so for the developing countries like India have come out of long suppressive rule and gained their freedom for independent socio-economic development. Health care is an important part of these programmes. Since vast majority of the population live in rural India, rural health care assures added importance.

Since the attainment of independence the country made a significant progress in improving the health status of its people through national programmes such as National Small Pox Eradication Programme, the Malaria Eradication Programme and Tuberculosis Control Programmes etc. As a result of various national programmes, the death rates in the population declined sharply during the period 1945-70 and the pace of decline in the death rates slowed down thereafter. Inspite of such impressive progress, the demographic and health picture of the country still constitutes a cause for serious and urgent concern. The high rate of population growth continues to have an adverse effect on the health of the people and the quality of their lives. The mortality rate for women and children are distressingly high, almost one-third of total deaths occur among the children below the age 5; infant mortality rate is around 129 per 1000 live birth. All the prevailing policies by the government has provided benefits to the upper crust of the society specially those residing in urban areas. It is imperative, therefore, that wherever the rural health programme have not taken root, a beginning is made by according priority for strengthening the existing health departments, promoting community health by provision of medicines and services through primary health care system. Hence, the Government of India initiated rural health schemes—namely Multipurpose Workers Schedule, Minimum Needs Programme, Village Health Guide Scheme, Maternity and Child Health Scheme, Universal Immunisation Programme etc. around 1975. It would be appropriate to examine how far the rural health programmes have influenced the demographic aspects. Keeping this in view an attempt has been made in this data to study for changes occurred in demographic variable in rural area during the period 1975-87. This paper is divided into three sections.

The first section contains a brief review of the health programmes in general and particularly in rural health programmes. In the second section the demographic changes that occurred in rural India are examined, and the third section deals with the feasibility of achieving the goal of 'Health for all by 2000 A.D.' for the country and also rural India.

REVIEW OF THE HEALTH PROGRAMMES

In this section, a brief review has been made regarding the the country's progress on public health and medical care system in general and in particularly among rural areas.

In 1946, the Heath Survey and Development Committee (Popularly known as Bhore Committee) had recommended to provide preventive, promotive and basic curative health service to all the citizens through a country wide not work of primary health centres and sub-centres. The recommendations were accepted and implemented immediately soon after independence. It was planned to have one primary health centre for every community block in rural areas of approximately for every 100000 population and sub-centres for every 30000 population.

Although the Government have accepted in principle the Bhore's Committee recommendations it was latter thought that, it would take a long time to implement all the recommendations, so the Government established national vertical programmes for the control of communicable disease such as Small pox, Tuberculosis, Malaria, Filaria and Leprosy etc.

Later the Government of India had set up a Health Survey and Planning Committee in 1959 (Mudaliar Committee) to review the developments in Public health and medical care that had taken place since independence and also formulation of all the recommendations for future plan of health development in the country. The Mudaliar Committee has recommended to recruit para-medical personnel for multi-purpose instead of individual diseases such as BCG, Leprosy, Malaria etc. and also recommended integration of medical and health services.

The national programmes in the field of Health and Family Planning and Nutrition were being run almost independently of each other by the staff recruited under each programme. There was no coordination between the field workers and supervisory staff of these programmes. Each national programme was conceived to run vertically with its staff. A committee on Multipurpose workers under Health and Family Planning Programme (also known as Kartar Singh Committee) was appointed by the Government of India to find out whether the same objectives could be achieved by coordinating the national programme and pooling the personal. The committee recommended that the multipurpose workers for the delivery of Health and Family Planning and Nutrition services are both feasible and desirable. The Committee also recommended the integration at different levels. The doctors at PHC's should render health care to the population and also should check the work of health workers at the sub-centres and their supervisors.

The minimum needs programmes concept was introduced in the 5th Five Year Plan, with the idea that it would be the main instrument through which health infrastructure in rural areas would be expanded and further strengthened to ensure primary health care to the rural population. The minimum needs programme was supported by the centrally sponsored schemes of community health volunteers, and Reorientation of Medical education were initiated in 1977. The community health volunteers programme had the objective of providing a trained community health volunteer selected by the community itself for every village or a population of 1000. The Reorientation of Medical Education Scheme was initiated with the twin objective of providing curative health care facilities to the rural people and giving a rural bias to medical education.

The country has adopted the policy of 'Health for all by 2000 AD' enunciated in Alma Ata Declaration in 1978. The health system in the country has to be restructured and re-oriented towards these policy projective and measures have to be initiated to correct regional imbalances' prevalent within the system.

During the Sixth plan, National Health policy was adopted in 1983 by both houses of parliament. Health Care programmes were restructured and reoriented towards this policy. Priority was given to extension of rural health infrastructure through a net work of community health centres, primary health centres and subcentres in a liberalised norm.

While it was the general situation, in rural areas the prevailing Health Schemes are—Minimum Need Programme, Multipurpose workers scheme, Community Health Voluntary Programme and Maternal and Child Health Supplementary Programme. Let us now discuss these schemes in detail.

Minimum Need Programme

One of the most important components of Minimum Need Programmes is the Rural Health Programme. It has been agreed in principle that under the Minimum Need Programme the objective to be achieved in phased manner through a successive plan period by 2000 would be as follows :

(a) One sub-centres with one male and one female Multipurpose Health Worker for every 5000 rural population and 3000 in tribal and hilly areas.

(b) One Primary Health Centres for every 30000 rural population (2000 population in tribal and hilly areas)

(c) One Community Health Centres/Upgraded PRC for over one lakh population with 30 beds.

(d) One village heatlh guide for every village for an average of 1000 rural population.

(e) One trained dai for every village.

As on 31st December 1987, 14,009 primary health centres and 102,674 subcentres are functioning. The number of PHC has increased from 7284 in December 1985 to 14609 in 1987. While the sub-centres has increased from 84,590 in 1985 to 102674 in 1987. The number of community Health Centres were 1253 as on January 1988.

Multipurpose Workers Scheme

The multipurpose workers schemes was launched in 1974 with an aim of establishing a Health Delivery System through a team of multipurpose workers with one male and one female for every 5000 rural population. Implementation involved intensive training programme to train all existing purpose workers. As on 1-4-88 training was completed in 349 districts.

Village Health Guide Scheme

The Community Health volunteers scheme was introduced in the country on 2nd October 1977 with the objective of training a local person selected by the Community for Primary Health Care. On an average one person per 1000 rural or a village, was trained for three months.

Maternal & Child Health Supplementary Programme

One of the important aspects of the Health and Family Welfare Programme is the promotion of health of mothers and children. Under the basic MCH services, the health care for mothers and children was provided. The expanded programme of Immunization was started by the Government of India in 1978, with the objective of reducing morbidity, mortality and disabilities due to Diptheria, Portusis, Tetanus, Poliomyelitis, etc. In order to step up the pace of implementation of immunization scheme, Government started a special programme called 'Universal Immunization in 1985-86' with an objective of immunizing 85% of eligible infants against six vaccine preventable diseases and to protect 100% of pregnant women against tetanus. This programme was taken up in a phased manner in selected districts and catchment areas of medical colleges. It is proposed to extend the programme throughout the country by 1990. The catchment areas of 106 medical colleges have already been covered under the programme.

HEALTH PROGRAMMES : ITS IMPACT ON DEMOGRAPHIC VARIABLES

In this section an attempt has been made to study the changes occurred in the demographic variables in India since its independence, and particularly in rural areas from 1971 onwards. The information needed for proper assessment of the impact of public health and medical care on the morbidity and mortality levels of the population, particularly morbidity is grossly inadequate. The improvements in public health and medical care would have an immediate and direct effect on morbidity and the changes in morbidity would in turn influence mortality. Unfortunately the morbidity data is so poor both in coverage and in quality so no attempt has been made to analyses and compare it with public health programmes. Although vital events are collected through civil registration system from a century, still the registration of births and deaths are grossly under-registered. Only around 50 per cent of births and deaths are registered and there is no improvement since independence. The estimates of the mortality and fertility rates till the year 1971 are estimated from various censuses. But the information related to the CBR & CDR, were not available separately for rural and urban areas till 1971. Since 1968, Sample Registration Scheme has been initiated in the country. The estimates of birth and death rates based in Sample Registration System have been published yearly by state-wise and for the urban and rural areas separately. Hence the SRS data is used for this paper which is considered to be reliable and accurate from the other sources.

With the SRS data an attempt has been made to study whether there exists an influence/impact on demographic variable due to improvements in public health and medical care. Therefore, to examine this relationship., the following demographic valuables are selected.

1. Population composition for rural India for the period 1961-81.
2. Mortality indicators
3. Age specific death rates in rural India.
4. Distribution of deaths by age group.
5. Distribution of deaths by major cause group.

Composition of Rural Population

Let us first examine the composition of rural population by age group and changes that occurred in India. Two important observations have emerged from Table 1. Children aged 0-4 years accounted for 15.36% of the total population in 1961 decreased to 14.9 in 1971 and further reduced to 12.89 in 1981. This change can be mainly attributed to reduction in fertility i.e. by increase in the family planning acceptance rate and reduction in infant mortality Table 1 further shows that the proportion of people aged 60 and above increased from less than 6%

of the total population in 1961 to about 7% in 1981. Eradication or control of a communicable diseases are partly responsible for the increase in the proportion of people aged 60 and above over the years.

Table 1 : Percentage distribution of population by age groups in Rural areas

Age-groups	*1961*	*1971*	*1981*
0-4	15.36	14.91	12.89
5-14	26.12	27.85	27.61
15-44	42.24	40.58	41.75
45-59	10.42	10.42	10.87
60+	5.83	6.23	6.84
Total	100.00	100.00	100.00

Source : Registrar General of India, Census of India, Social Cultural Tables : 1961, 1971 and 1981.

Mortality indicators

Table 2 provides data on trends in selected indicators of mortality levels in India. It shows that, there has been a substantial and steady decline during the period 1951-71 and the pace of death rates in the population have declined there after and was staggering around a value of 15 for the period 1973-78. Since 1978, the decline has considerably slowed down and in 1987 and death rate is estimated at 10.8% thousand population per year. The sharp decline in death rates during the period 1951-71 is mainly due to the improvements in public health and medical care programmes, particularly due to various national programmes on controlling communicable diseases rather than improvement in socio-economic conditions of the people. In order to bring down the crude death rates it is not just sufficient only to control the communicable diseases but also necessary to reduce the levels of infant and child mortality.

The infant mortality rate or the deaths of children below one year of age, are generally related to 1000 live births. The infant mortality rate has declined rapidly from a level of 146 for the decade 1951-1961 to 129 for the decade 1961-71. Like CDR the level of IMR was houring around 130 for the period 1966-77. Since 1978, there appears to be decline in the level of infant mortality rate and in 1987; the Infant mortality rate is estimated to be 95.

Table 2 : Mortality Indicators, 1976 to 1987 All India

Year	*Crude death rate*	*Infant mortality rate*	*Neo-natal mortality rate*	*Post-natal mortality rate*	*Peri-natal mortality rate*
1	*2*	*3*	*4*	*5*	*6*
			RURAL		
1976	16.3	139.0	83.0	56.28	76.6
1977	16.0	140.0	88.0	52.0	69.5
1978	15.3	137.0	85.2	51.8	67.9
1979	13.9	129.7	77.7	52.0	63.1
1980	13.5	123.8	75.5	48.3	59.8
1981	13.7	119.1	75.6	43.5	58.8
1982	13.1	113.7	72.9	40.8	57.7
1983	13.1	113.8	73.6	40.2	57.7
1984	13.8	113.8	72.2	41.4	58.3
1985	13.0	107.0	66.6	39.9	52.4
1986	12.2	105.0	-	-	-
1987	11.9	104.0	-	-	-
			URBAN		
1976	9.5	80.0	49.0	31.17	43.7
1977	9.4	81.0	42.0	39.0	35.4
1978	9.4	74.0	38.0	36.0	33.5
1979	8.4	72.2	42.1	29.8	38.7
1980	8.0	65.2	38.1	26.1	35.3
1981	7.8	62.5	38.5	24.0	31.5
1982	7.4	65.2	38.8	26.4	33.1
1983	7.9	65.8	39.3	26.5	35.4
1984	8.6	66.1	39.7	26.4	35.7

1985	7.8	59.0	38.3	25.6	50.4
1986	7.6	62.0	-	-	-
1987	7.3	61.0	-	-	-
			COMBINED		
1976	15.0	129.0	77.0	52.0	66.8
1977	14.7	130.0	80.2	49.8	63.7
1978	14.2	127.0	77.4	49.6	62.2
1979	12.8	120.0	71.7	48.3	59.0
1980	12.4	113.9	69.3	44.6	55.7
1981	12.5	110.4	69.9	40.5	54.6
1982	11.9	104.8	66.7	38.1	53.2
1983	11.9	104.9	68.2	37.7	53.6
1984	12.6	104.0	65.8	38.2	53.8
1985	11.8	97.0	60.1	37.1	48.1
1986	11.1	96.0	-	-	-
1987	10.8	95.0	-	-	-

Source : Registrar General, India-Sample Registration System.

The table reveals that both the crude death rates and infant mortality rates for the rural areas have always been significantly higher than in urban areas. One of the possible reasons for this difference can be attributed to the better health and medical facilities that are available in urban areas than in the rural areas. In the year 1988, the number hospitals and dispensaries in rural urban areas are 16308, 21009 respectively. This clearly indicates that how the medical and public health facilities are disproportionately higher, in urban areas interms of the population, than in the rural areas. It is gratifying to note that both in urban and in rural areas the crude death rates and infant mortality rates showed a sharp decline from 1978 onwards. In rural areas the crude death rates have declined from 16.3 in 1976 to 11.9 in 1987, while infant mortality rates have reduced from 140 in 1976 to 104 in 1987. On the other hand in urban areas the respective crude death rate and infant mortality rates in the year 1976 were 9.5 and 80 and these rates have reduced sharply to 7.3 and 61. The sharp reduction in crude death rates and infant mortality rates particularly in rural areas from 1977 may partly be attributed to the introduction of the rural health schemes namely minimum needs programme, multipurpose worker schemes, maternal and child health services and health guide schemes. But it is extremely difficult to pinpoint exactly the contribution of public health programme in bringing down the changes in mortality rates as the socio-economic development would also contribute for the reduction.

The neo-natal and post natal mortality rates in 1977 were 77 and 52 respectively, and the corresponding rates have come down to 60 and 37 in the year 1985. A significant difference between rural and urban areas have noticed in all the years between neonatal and post natal mortality rates. In both rural and in urban areas neo-natal as well post neonatal rates have reduced considerably from the year 1977 onwards.

The perinatal mortality also showed more or less similar trend as it was observed with respect to neo-natal and post-natal mortality. In general, it can be pointed out that, the reduction in IMR, neo-natal mortality, and post natal mortality are mainly due to the implementation of MCH activities in rural as well as in urban areas. Even in 1986, 60% of infant mortality occurs in the first 28 days or perinatal period, and is largely a result of factors that are not very difficult to avoid. Hence for lowering the infants mortality in a significant manner, the highest priority should be given (to services for child births and care for the new born) appropriately to perinatal care including immunisation against tetanus which can reduce infant mortality by at least 50% or so.

Proportion of deaths

Table 3 provides data on the percentage of deaths by age group in rural India in selected years. A number of interesting observations can be made from this table. Infant deaths which accounted for 22.4% of the total deaths in 1968 have gradually but steadily reduced to 16.3 in 1986. Similarly, deaths among children 1-4 years have been reduced from 14.2 in 1968 to 8.3 in 1987. Deaths among children aged 5-14 years have been reduced considerably from 6.4% of the total deaths in 1968 to 4.8% in 1983. The decline in infant and child mortality rates may be due to various reasons, important among them are improvements in public health and medical care and provision of more and better maternal and child health services. The proportion of deaths among those aged 15-54 years showed a marginal increase of about one per cent during the period 1968-1986. It is striking to note from the table 2 that the proportion of deaths among those age 55 years and over has increased from 35.7% of deaths in 1968 to 46.8% in 1986. The pausible reason for this increase is due to.

Table 3 : Percentage distribution of deaths by age group in rural India in selected years

Age - Groups	*1968*	*1973*	*1978*	*1983*	*1986*
Below 1	22.4	20.3	19.2	16.8	16.3
1-4	14.2	12.3	9.9	7.8	8.3
5-14	6.4	6.5	5.3	4.6	4.8
15-34	9.4	9.8	9.2	9.8	10.9
35-54	11.9	12.7	12.7	12.8	12.9
54 +	35.7	38.4	43.7	48.2	46.8
Total	100.00	100.00	100.00	100.00	100.00

Source : Registrar General of India : *'Causes of Death—A survey'* vital Registration Division New Delhi.

(a) increase in the proportion of people aged 55 years and over

(b) The proportion of deaths among children to total deaths has been decreasing. So the proportion of deaths among these aged 55 years have been increasing.

In order to over come this artifact, the age specific death rates have been studied. Table 4 provides data on age specific death rates for rural areas in India. It is evident from the table that the age specific death rates have declined for all the age groups during the period 1972-85 particularly among the children aged 0-4 years. The age specific death rates for the age group 0-4 has steadily declined from 62.7 in 1972 to 43.3 in 1985. Similarly the age specific death rates for the people aged 70 and above has reduced from 133.3 in 1972 to 100 in 1985. In rural areas, the age specific death rates for males were lower than females upto the age group 30-34 and the picture became reverse from the subsequent age groups. One of the significant points emerged from the table is, in rural areas, the age specific death rates between male and female were more among the age groups 15-19, 20-

24, 25-29 and 30-34. This may be partly due to the prevalence of maternal mortality in these age groups. It is interesting to observe that for urban areas, the female showed a higher age specific death rates (though gap was more among rural as compared to urban areas) than males in the age groups 15-19 and 20-24 years. Unfortunately maternal mortality statistics for urban and rural areas are not available separately. At the same time from the Table 4, it indicates that it is required to improve MCH activities more in rural areas to reduce IMR and maternal mortality rates.

Table 4 : Age Specific Death Rates in Rural India : 1972-85

Age Group	*Years*					
	1972	*1976*	*1980*	*1985*		
				Persons	*Males*	*Females*
0-4	62.7	55.2	46.1	41.4	45.3	43.3
5-9	5.9	5.2	4.0	3.7	4.8	4.2
10-14	2.5	2.6	1.8	2.0	2.1	2.0
15-19	3.3	2.9	2.7	2.0	3.1	2.6
20-24	4.6	3.7	3.3	2.8	4.2	3.5
25-29	4.7	4.3	3.4	3.1	4.1	3.6
30-34	5.4	5.0	3.7	3.5	4.4	3.9
35-39	6.1	5.1	5.0	4.3	4.2	4.3
40-44	8.7	7.4	6.6	7.2	5.4	6.4
45-49	11.6	9.7	8.8	10.2	7.3	8.8
50-54	17.8	16.6	13.1	15.0	11.1	13.2
55-59	26.4	24.1	19.8	23.1	16.3	19.8
60-64	42..8	42.8	32.2	37.4	28.4	32.9
65-69	62.3	53.0	52.6	50.6	40.2	95.3
70+	133.3	101.6	94.0	106.2	94.2	100.1
All ages	18.9	16.3	13.5	12.9	13.1	13.0

Source : Directorate General of Health Services, Hand Book Health Information, India 1988.

Causes of Death

It is very difficult to obtain in surveys the information on causes of deaths in India because a majority of the deaths occur in home and not in the hospital. As the majority of people are illiterate, they are usually ignorant about the cause of death. The situation has improved in recent years due to the introduction of Model Registration Scheme or Survey of cause of Death which is collecting information on causes of death in rural areas of the country. The data are collected by paramedics attached to the primary health centres. Table 5 provides the data on the percentage distribution of deaths by major cause groups for the rural areas of the country in 1970, 75, 78, 80 and 86. The interesting points that are emerged from the table are that in 1975, the 'cough group diseases claimed the highest percentage of deaths with 21.1% and the 'senility' group accounted for 16.8% of deaths. Fevers and causes peculiar to infancy had contributed 13 and 12.5% of total deaths. There was a significant increase in the percentage of deaths due to 'senility' and it increased from 16.8 in 1970 to 22.4 in 1986. The proportion of deaths due to 'cough' had fluctuated around 20% through out the period. It may be mentioned that 'Diseases of circulatory system' and other clear symptoms contributed between 7 to 9% of total deaths. The percentage of' 'Accident of injuries' had increased from 4.6% of deaths in 1975 due to 7.0% of deaths in 1986. A further insight can be gained by examining the changing pattern of the incidence of death by cause groups. Deaths due to the 'cough' (Disorders of the respiratory system) occupied the first rank in 1975 and 1976 but in 1980, 1983, 1986, they were pushed down to second rank. Deaths due to 'senility' which occupied second rank in 1975 improved to the first rank in 1978, 1980 and 1983. Deaths due to 'Digestive disorders' and 'cause peculiar to infancy' occupied third and fourth ranks in 1985 and the positions were reversed in 1936. This table clearly indicates the deaths due to 'causes peculiar to infancy' had reduced dramatically over a period of time and this a mainly due to improvements in MCH and immunisation programmes from 1978 on wards. Deaths due to 'senility' has increased over a period of time which is mainly because of the eradication or control of communicable diseases and also due to the old age diseases that have registered an increase over a period of time.

Table 5 : Percentage distribution of deaths by major cause groups in Rural India for selected years

Major cause groups (Prominent symptoms)	*1975*	*1978*	*1980*	*1983*	*1986*
1. Accident and injuries	4.6 (8)	4.9 (8)	5.0 (8)	5.5 (8)	7.0 (8)
2. Child birth & Pregnancy	1.0 (11)	1.0 (11)	1.2 (11)	1.2 (10)	1.0 (10)
3. Fevers	13.2 (3)	9.6 (4)	8.5 (6)	10.2 (4)	10.4 (4)
4. Digestive Disorders	9.8 (5)	9.3 (5)	9.3 (4)	7.4 (6)	7.7 (7)
5. Coughs (Disorders of respiratory system)	21.1 (1)	20.6 (1)	20.0 (2)	20.2 (2)	19.7 (2)
6. Disorders of the central nervous system	3.2 (10)	3.6 (9)	3.8 (9)	4.5 (9)	3.7 (9)
7. Diseases of circulatory system	7.0 (7)	9.0 (6)	8.6 (5)	9.1 (5)	9.0 (5)
8. Other clear symptoms	7.4 (6)	7.8 (7)	7.5 (7)	7.4 (6)	8.6 (6)
9. Causes peculiar to infancy	12.5 (4)	13.0 (3)	13.6 (3)	11.0 (3)	10.5 (3)
10. Senility	16.8 (2)	19.2 (2)	20.7 (1)	23.2 (1)	22.4
11. The rest	3.4 (9)	2.0 (10)	1.8 (10)	0.3 (11)	- -
All Causes	100.00	100.00	100.00	100.00	100.00

Notes : Figures in the parenthesis notes the ranks

Source : Office of the Registrar General, India, Various, SRs, Survey Report, Registrar General, Newsletter.

Future Perspectives

In order to achieve the goal of 'Health for all by 2000 AD' the experts have drawn a long term objective, of population stabilisation by Net Reproductive Rate (NRR) to 1 by 2000. Along with the objective of achieving NRR=1, the goals are also fixed for other crucial variables such as CDR, CBR, IMR, Expectation of life at births (Years). Effective couple protection rate, percentage of pregnant mothers receiving ante natal care and Immunization status etc., and these are shown in Table 6. It would be desirable to take stock of the present levels of those crucial variables and see the existing gaps between the goals and achievement.

Crude Death Rate : The crude death rate of India for the year 1987 is estimated to be 10.8 and respective rates for urban and rural areas were 11.9 and 7.3 respectively. Urban areas have already achieved less than the goal of 9 CDR fixed for 2000 AD. Only the rural areas are lagging behind. There is wide regional disparity between the states with respect to CDRs for instance, the crude death rates for the states (in rural areas) of U.P., Bihar, Madhya Pradesh and Orissa are more than 13. It is gratifying to note that the CDR in U.P. has registered a sharp decline from 19.1 in 1980 to 15.3 in 1987. It would be possible to achieve the goal of CDR to 9 by 2000 A.D. particularly for rural areas of Uttar Pradesh, Bihar, Madhya Pradesh and Rajasthan only if intensive efforts have been done for strengthening and utilizing the primary health care services.

Infant Mortality Rate : The infant mortality rate for India as a whole is estimated to be 95 in 1987 and the respective urban and rural rates were 59 and 104. It would be extremely difficult to achieve the target of 60 (IMR) by 2000 AD for rural areas of India is general and particularly for the states of Uttar Pradesh, Orissa, and Madhya Pradesh whose rates were 135, 130 and 127 respectively. The infant mortality rates in rural areas of India have reduced substantially and steadily from 124 in 1980 to 104 in 1987. Similarly in U.P., The IMR, for rural areas had shown a sharp reduction from 167 in 1980 to 135 in 1987. The reduction in IMR particularly in Rural areas from 1980 onwards may be mainly contributed by the initiation of the expanded programme of immunization (EPI) from 1977 onwards.

In addition to the universal immunisation programme the supply of safe drinking water to rural areas also brought down infant and childhood mortality at a faster rate. Maternal and child health programmes play a major role to reduce morbidity and mortality particularly infant mortality. All the items included in EPI programme

Table 6 : Goals for Health and Family Welfare Programmes

Sl. No.	*Indicator*	*Current Level*	*Goals 1985*	*Goals 1990*	*Goals 2000*
1	2	*3*	*4*	*5*	*6*
1.	Infant mortality rate				
	Rural	104 (1987)*	122		
	Urban	61 (1987)*	60		
	Total	95 (1987)*	106	87	below 60
	Perinatal mortality	48.1 (1985)			30-35
2.	Crude death rate	10.8 (1987)*	12	10.4	9.0
3.	Pre-school child (1-5 years) mortality	24 (1976-77)	20-24	15.20	10
4.	Maternal mortality rate	4-5 (1976)	3-4	2-3	below 2
5.	Life Expectancy at Birth (Years)				
	Male	52.6 (1976-81) 55.6 (1981-86)	55.1	57.6	61
	Female	51.6 (1976-81) 56.4 (1981-86)	54.3	57.1	64
6.	Babies with birth weight below 2500 gms (percentage)	30	25	18	10
7.	Crude birth rate	3200 (1987)*	31	29.1	21.0
8.	Effective·couple protection rate (Percentage)	23.7 (March, 82) 39.8 (March, 88)	37.0	42.0	60.0

9.	Net Reproduction Rate (NRR)	1.48 (1981)	1.34	1.17	1.00
10.	Growth Rate (annual)	2.28 (1971-81)	1.90	1.66	1.20
11.	Family Size	4.4 (1975)	3.8		2.3
12.	Pregnant mothers receiving ante-natal care (%)	40-50	50-60	60-75	100
13.	Deliveries by trained birth attendants (%)	30.35	50	580	100
14.	Immunisations status (% coverage)				
	TT (for Pregnant women)	57.49 (1937-88)	60	100	100
	10 Years	20	40	100	100
	16 years	20	60	100	100
	DPT (children below 3 years)	72.62 (1987-88)	70	85	85
	Polio (infants)	63.14 (1987-88)	50	70	85
	BCG (infants)	71.19 (1987-88)	70	80	85
	DT (new school entrants 5-6 years)	20	80	85	85
	Typhoid (new school entrants 5-6 years)	2	70	85	85
15.	Leprosy-percentage of disease arrested cases out of those detected	20	40	60	80
16.	TB-percentage of diseases arrested cases out of those detected	50	60	75	90
17.	Blindness-incidence of (%)	1.4	1	0.7	0.3

Source : National Health Policy Document

*Provisional

such as TT (PN), DPT, Polio, BCG, Measles, ET, Typohid TT (10 years,) TTP (6 years,) achieved between 90-95 per cent of the target fixed in the year 1987-88. If the programme continue in the same manner it would be able to achieve the goals by 2000 AD.

SUGGESTIONS TO STRENGHTEN HEALTH CARE SERVICES

The norms fixed for the establishment of PHCs and Subcentres are based on population through out the country (though there are some minor modifications in tribal and hilly areas). The average size of village in Kerala was 16967 in 1981; 966 in Bihar and 808 in Uttar Pradesh. It is obvious than there will be subcentres located in the villages in Kerala. The access of the people to primary health care would be greater in Kerala state than in U.P. or Bihar. Another dimension of the problem is the physical accessibility. In Kerala, for every 100 sq. kms the length of road was 275 sq. cm. On the other hand the imparable figures for Bihar, Madhya Pradesh and Rajasthan were 48, 24 and 21 respectively. In Kerala 100% of villages are linked with roads and the comparable figures for Bihar and U.P. were 39 and 25%. It is also found in a study that smaller the village, is, lower the accessibility and vice versa. The administrators and policy makers should consider the physical accessibility as an important factor in planning for primary health care.

It is necessary to conduct in depth studies at frequent intervals to know the utilization of primary health centres and subcentres.

Since independence the Government of India and various State Governments have launched a number of public health and medical care programmes in the country for improving the health and longevity of the people. The mortality rate has declined from 27.4 in 1941-51 to an estimated 10.8 in 1987. The expectation of life at birth has gone up from about 32 years during 1941-51 to about 50.5 years during 1971-81. The infant mortality has come down from 140 in 1975 to 95 in 1987. Further the health infrastructure facilities has been strengthened for the welfare of the people. The country has about 14609 Primary Health Centres, and 102674 Subcentres as on 31-12-87. The per capita expenditure on health incurred by the state has gone up from about Rs. 1.50 in 1955-56 to about 46.23 Rs. in 1985-86.

There is significant difference between rural and urban areas with respect to CDR, IMR, etc. The infant mortality rates for rural and urban areas in the year 1971 were 138 and 82 respectively and the corresponding figures for the year 1987 were 104 and 61.

The infant mortality rate and CDR has come down considerably from 1978 onwards particularly in rural areas. This may be accounted partly due to the introduction of Minimum Need Programme, MCH and expanded immunisation programme. The vital rates and infant mortality rate varies widely among the states. The crude death rates and infant mortality rates for Kerala state in the year 1987 were estimate to be 6.0 and while the corresponding rates for U.P. state were 14.3 and 126. The gap between rural and urban areas were more among the underdeveloped states such as Uttar Pradesh, Bihar, Madhya Pradesh and Rajasthan, on the other hand, the gap was narrowed among the developed states such as Kerala.

If the country has to achieve the goal of 'Health for all by 2000 AD' it is very much essential to make substantial efforts towards the promotion of primary health care services in rural areas, particularly more so in rural areas of the under developed states.

ACKNOWLEDGEMENTS

The author is grateful to Mr. S. Surender for his valuable assistance throughout the preparation of paper.

REFERENCES

1. Bose, A., "Logistic support and facilities for primary health care : The crucial role of physical accessibility", *Proceedings of the Seminar, Health for All, Concept and Reailty,* (Ed) Sanya Gill, Bombay, 1985.
2. Directorate General of Health Services, India, *Health Information India-1988,* New Delhi.
3. Directorate General of Health Services, India, Health *Services in India,* 1981-82, New Delhi, 1988.
4. Directorate General of Health Services, India, *Hand Book of Health Information of India, New Delhi, 1988.*
5. Family Welfare Programme in India, Year Book 1974-75 to 1987-88, New Delhi.
6. Government of India, *Sixth Five Year Plan 1980-85, New Delhi.*
7. Government of India, Seventh Five Year Plan 1985-90, New Delhi.
8. *Health for All : An Alternative Strategy,* Report of a study group, set up jointly by the Indian Council of Social science research and the Indian Council of Medical Research, New Delhi, August 1980.

9. Lok Sabha Secretariat, India, National *Health Policy,* New Delhi, 1989.
10. Office of the Registrar General, India, *Causes of Death (Rural)* 1973-88, A Survey, New Delhi.
11. Reddy, P.H., "Epidemiologic transition in India", Population transition in India (Eds.) S.H. Singh et. al., B.R. Publishing Corporation, New Delhi, 1989.
12. Registrar General of India, *Sample Registration System, 1987,* New Delhi.

8

A NOTE ON MORTALITY AND MORBIDITY IN ANDHRA PRADESH

Prof. G. Ramachandrudu

INTRODUCTION

It has become common place to observe that as mortality falls, morbidity levels rise. The plausible explanations for this dichotomous phenomenon are given by Ryan Johansson (1991) and Gopalakrishna Kumar (1993). The urban areas, which are known for lower mortality rates, logically must be having a higher morbidity levels when compared to rural areas. Unfortunately, the data on morbidity in India are so inadequate to make out any scientific analysis. Existence of disproportionately large medical and health facilities available in urban areas should not be considered as an index of better health status, infact it could be the opposite. Also the urban medical and health facilities are being used by large number of rural people as well. In Andhra Pradesh the increasing rural to urban migration caused by the rapid changes in agriculture (for ex : Farmers are shifting from agriculture to pisciculture in Coastal region which require less labour) could also lead to increasing morbidity in urban areas especially in slums and squatter settlements (Rao B.S. and Ramachandrudu G., 1991). The Objective of this note is to analyse the mortality and morbidity data available in Andhra Pradesh.

HEALTH INFORMATION SYSTEMS IN INDIA

Management of Health information systems is an essential tool for the provision of insights into the planning, administration and improving the quality of health services in a given area. The Primary objective of collecting and processing data at the grassroot level should be to facilitate decision making, for field workers and the community at large. Information gathered may be passed on to the middle and higher levels of administration to aid policy decisions. At the community level, information should be utilised for self monitoring and establishing priorities. In India, unfortunately, most of the programme administrators do not feel that they need statistical information, probably because the facts are stranger than fiction. Even this inadequate health information reveals quite a bit of insights into the health practices of our masses.

Presently there are about seven sources of health information in India. These are :

(a) Decennial Population Census

(b) Civil Registration System (CRS)

(c) Sample Registration System (SRS)

(d) Survey of causes of death

(e) National Sample Survey (NSS)

(f) Family Welfare Statistics

(g) Management Information and Evaluation System (MIES)

In addition, each national health programme has its own system of collecting and analysing programme specific data, some more sophisticated than others, but all of which function independently. Thus there are several parallel flows of information and it is virtually impossible to get a total picture of any particular district, leave alone the entire country. During early 1980s, as a result of the recommendations of expert groups, a new system of integrated records was implemented in various states. This system specified the minimum number of records to be maintained to cover essential information. Information collected by the Primary Health Centres (PHCs) would be passed to the Centre through the district health departments, and returned to the districts after the information was processed. This elaborate strategy failed for various reasons. Recently, the Central Bureau of Health Intelligence (CBHI) in the Ministry of Health and Family Welfare established an integrated Management Information and Evaluation System (MIES) for the entire health and family planning programme in the country. Under this scheme, the PHC is expected to forward information of its various activities, which is to eventually reach the CBHI in the form of reports for computerisation and generation of output tables. Non-availability of adequately trained statistical staff at the Primary Health Centres the future of such a system seems bleak.

The Civil Registration System (CRS) which attempts to collect information on birth and deaths, suffers from incomplete Coverage and under-Registration. In the absence of dependable vital rates from civil registration, the office of the Registrar General, initiated the Sample Registration System (SRS) in 1964-65 on a pilot basis and on full scale from 1969-70. This is a demographic sample survey based on a dual record system. The field investigation under Sample Registration System consists of continuous enumeration of births and deaths in a sample of villages/urban blocks by a resident part-time enumerator, and an independent six monthly retrospective survey by a full-time supervisor. The data obtained through these two sources are matched and unmatched events will be cross checked. Thus, the SRS is providing fairly reliable estimates of the vital events for the country as well as for the states. However, the SRS could not provide the estimates at the district level. In Andhra Pradesh, there are 190 rural sample units (villages) and 100 urban sample units (blocks) and the Directorate of Census Operations and the Directorate of Health are Organising the SRS.

The Office of the Registrar General, conducts Survey of Causes of Death (Rural) ever since in 1982. In Andhra Pradesh the survey is being conducted in 82 Primary Health Centres. The survey is confined to headquarter village only. This is done by trained para-medical staff.

TRENDS IN MORTALITY IN A.P.

The dimensions of health improvement and mortality decline have been assessed under the conceptual framework of "health transition" by a number of analysts, largely influenced by the work of John Caldwell (1989). He suggested that the health transition should be seen as an extension of the "epidemiological transition" a concept that relates to changing patterns in the causes of deaths. The simultaneous decline of infectious diseases and rise in chronic diseases in populations experiencing mortality declines has spawned numerous efforts to explain how and why health improves in diverse populations. Many of these contributions emphasize and synergism between medical and biological variables on the one hand and the socio-economic context in which these operate on the other (Ryan Johansson, 1991). In this section, we analyse the recent trends in mortality in India and

Andhra Pradesh with special reference to urban areas of Andhra Pradesh.

Table 1 presents trends in crude death rates in All India and Andhra Pradesh during 1981-92. The crude death rate in India fell from 12.1 in 1981-83 to 9.8 in 1990-92, a decline of 19 per cent. On the other hand the Crude Death Rate (CDR) in Andhra Pradesh fell from 10.7 to 9.3, that is, by 13 per cent during the corresponding period. The rate of decline in rural areas in much higher in both India and Andhra Pradesh. What is more significant in this mortality transition is that in Andhra Pradesh, both in the rural as well as urban areas, there is a slower rate of transition when compared to all India. Infact, urban rate of mortality decline in Andhra Pradesh in only one-third of All India (3.0 per cent as against 9.1 per cent).

Table 1 : Trends in Crude Death Rate in India and Andhra Pradesh (1981-92)

Period	*All India*				*Andhra Pradesh*			
	Combined (C)	*Rural (R)*	*Urban (U)*	*U/R*	*Combined (C)*	*Rural (R)*	*Urban (U)*	*U/R*
1981-83	12.1	13.3	7.7	0.58	10.7	11.7	6.7	0.57
1982-84	12.1	13.3	8.0	0.60	10.7	11.6	7.4	0.64
1983-85	12.1	13.3	8.1	0.61	10.5	11.3	7.7	0.68
1984-86	11.8	13.0	8.0	0.62	10.4	11.2	7.6	0.68
1985-87	11.3	12.4	7.6	0.61	10.0	10.8	7.2	0.67
1986-88	11.0	12.0	7.6	0.63	10.0	10.7	7.3	0.68
1987-89	10.7	11.7	7.4	0.64	9.9	10.6	7.2	0.68
1988-90	10.3	11.2	7.2	0.64	9.6	10.3	7.0	0.68
1989-91	9.9	10.7	7.1	0.66	9.4	10.2	6.7	0.66
1990-92	9.8	10.7	7.0	0.65	9.3	10.0	6.5	0.65
Percent Decline (1982-92)	19.0	19.5	9.1	-	13.1	14.5	3.0	-

Source : Registrar General, India—Sample Registration Bulletin Vol. 28, No. 1, Jan., 1994.

Table 1 also presents the urban-rural ratios of the Crude Death Rates. It can be observed from the table that the rural CDRs are higher than those of urban areas by about 30-40 per cent in both Andhra Pradesh as well as All India. It is interesting to note that almost all the ratios of Andhra Pradesh are higher than those of All India, indicating lesser rural and urban differentials in CDR. It can also be observed from the table that the urban-rural ratios in India as well as Andhra Pradesh are increasing over time indicating the narrowing down the gap between rural and urban mortality rates which may indicate a lower rate of improvement in health status in urban areas. In Andhra Pradesh, the ratio has increased from 0.57 during 1981-83 to a high of 0.68 by 1988-90 and then declined slightly to 0.65 in 1990-92.

Infant mortality rate has widely been recognised as a comprehensive index of socio-economic development as well as health status. Table 2 presents the trends in Infant Mortality Rate (IMR) for All India and Andhra Pradesh during 1981-92, by residence. The IMR for India has declined from a high of 107 per 1000 live births during 1981-83 to a low of 80 per 1000 during 1990-92, that is by 25 per cent, whereas for Andhra Pradesh, IMR has declined from 81 per 1000 live births to 70 per 1000 during the same period, that is, by 12 per cent. Thus the rate of decline in IMR in India was higher than that of Andhra Pradesh, partly because of relatively lower IMR in Andhra Pradesh than that of All India at the base period 1981-83.

Table 2 also presents the urban-rural differentials of the Infant Mortality Rate. Urban infant mortality rate in Andhra Pradesh has been rising from 52 per 1000 live births during 1981-83 to 61 per 1000 during 1984-86 and then declined to 55 per 1000 during 1989-91. This should be a matter of great concern to the health planners of the State. It can be observed from the table that rural IMRs are higher than those of urban areas by about the same extent as in the case of CDR (See Table 1). Once again, it is observed that all the ratios of Andhra Pradesh are higher than those of All India, indicating a lesser rural urban differentials in infant mortality rates. Same as in the case of CDR, the urban-rural ratios are increasing over the period 1981-92, indicating the narrowing down the gap between rural and urban areas. In Andhra Pradesh, the ratio has increased from 0.60 during 1981-83 to a high of 0.71 in 1984-86 and then declined to 0.68 in 1990-92.

Table 2 : Three year moving average of infant mortality rates of All India and Andhra Pradesh (1981-92)

Year	*All India*				*Andhra Pradesh*			
	Combined (C)	*Rural (R)*	*Urban (U)*	*U/R*	*Combined (C)*	*Rural (R)*	*Urban (U)*	*U/R*
1981-83	107	116	65	0.56	81	87	52	0.60
1982-84	105	114	66	0.58	78	83	57	0.69
1983-85	102	111	64	0.58	79	84	59	0.70
1984-86	99	108	62	0.57	81	86	61	0.71
1985-87	96	105	60	0.57	81	87	58	0.67
1986-88	94	104	61	0.59	81	87	60	0.69
1987-89	93	102	60	0.59	81	87	58	0.67
1988-90	88	96	57	0.59	78	83	57	0.69
1989-91	84	90	54	0.60	74	79	55	0.70
1990-92	80	86	52	0.61	71	76	52	0.68
Percent Decline (1982-92)	25.2	25.9	20.0	-	12.3	12.6	0.0	-

Source : Office of the Registrar General India—*"Sample Registration Bulletin"*, Vol. 28, No. 1, Jan., 1994.

Infant Mortality is influenced more by the reproductive health practices. The picture will be more clear if we look into more sophisticated measures of infant mortality. Table 3 presents certain mortality indicators by residence in All India and Andhra Pradesh. Neo-natal mortality rate (number of deaths below the age of 28 days per 1000 live births) in Andhra Pradesh (51) is much higher than that of All India (42), i.e. by 18 per cent. The urban neo-natal mortality rate in Andhra Pradesh (37) is 31 per cent higher than that of All India (25). This clearly shows reproductive health care in urban Andhra Pradesh is worse than that of All India. With regard to the urban post natal mortality, both Andhra Pradesh and All India figures are same. But wider variation is observed in urban peri-natal mortality as well as still birth rate. The urban peri-natal mortality rate (Number of deaths below the age of 7 days per 1000 live births) in Andhra Pradesh (47) is again larger than that of All India (26), i.e. by 45 per cent. The

Table 3 : Mortality indicators of All India and Andhra Pradesh (1991)

S. No.	*Indicator*	*All India*				*Andhra Pradesh*			
		Combined (C)	*Rural (R)*	*Urban (U)*	*U/R*	*Combined (C)*	*Rural (R)*	*Urban (U)*	*U/R*
1.	Neo-natal Mortality Rate	42.3	47.1	25.2	0.54	50.5	53.9	36.6	0.68
2.	Post-natal Mortality Rate	27.5	29.6	19.8	0.67	22.3	22.9	19.7	0.86
3.	Peri-natal Mortality Rate	39.7	43.5	25.8	0.59	55.9	58.2	46.8	0.80
4.	Still Birth Rate	10.9	11.8	7.5	0.64	14.7	13.8	18.5	1.34

* Excludes Jammu & Kashmir

Source : Sample Registration System (1991).

urban still birth rate (Number of still births per 1000 live births and still births) in Andhra Pradesh (19) is higher than that of All India (8), i.e. by 60 per cent. Surprisingly the still birth rate in urban areas (19) is higher than that of rural areas (14) in Andhra Pradesh. This indicates an alarming picture of reproductive health status in urban Andhra Pradesh.

Table 4 presents percentage distribution of specific causes of death under the group of causes peculiar to infancy for all India and Andhra Pradesh in 1986 and 1987. It can be observed from the table that prematurity is the most significant cause of infant death. In the country as a whole 44 per cent of deaths are due to prematurity in 1987, whereas the percentage in Andhra Pradesh is 36 per cent in 1986 and 24 per cent in 1987. While there is an increasing trend of this cause by 3 percentage points in India, there is sharp decline in this cause by 12 percentage points in Andhra Pradesh, and the other two major causes of infant deaths are respiratory infection and Diarrhoea (12 percent each). In Andhra Pradesh, almost all the classifiable causes of deaths are on the decline.

Table 4 : Percentage distribution of Specific causes under the group of causes peculiar to infancy for All India and Andhra Pradesh 1986 and 1987

S. No.	*Causes*	*All India*		*Andhra Pradesh*		*Change in Percentages*	
		1986	*1987*	*1986*	*1987*	*India*	*A.P.*
1.	Prematurity	41.0	43.9	36.0	24.2	2.9	-11.8
2.	Respiratory Infection	14.5	16.6	14.7	11.7	2.1	-3.0
3.	Diarrhoea of new born	10.2	10.0	4.0	11.7	-0.2	-7.7
4.	Cord Infection (including Tetanus)	7.7	6.9	2.6	2.1	-0.8	-0.5
5.	Congenital malformation	2.6	2.3	2.7	2.1	-0.3	-0.6
6.	Birth Injury	2.5	2.0	2.0	4.1	-0.5	2.1
7.	Not Classifiable specify symptom	21.5	18.3	38.0	44.1	-3.2	6.1
	Total	100.0	100.0	100.0	100.0		

A similar evidence is observed in the all India survey on infant and child mortality (1979). Table 5 presents top ten cause specific infant death rate per 10,000 children by sex in urban areas of Andhra Pradesh. In conformity with the evidence in Table 4, the all India Survey also has shown that prematurity is the most significant cause of infant death (about 10 per cent of children below one year die of prematurity) in Andhra Pradesh. About 4 per cent of children each die of tetanus and influenza. Another interesting observation of the data presented in the table is that measles among females is 7 times more prevalent than among males. Similarly malaria and infantile liver are 3 times more prevalent among females than males.

Table 5 : Top ten cause specific infant death rate per 10,000 Children by sex and residence in Andhra Pradesh (1978)

S. No.	*Causes*	*Urban*			
		Male (M)	*Female (F)*	*Person (P)*	*F/M*
1.	Prematurity	1448	539	966	0.37
2.	Tetanus	616	159	373	0.26
3.	Influenza	684	48	347	0.07
4.	Malaria	118	383	258	3.25
5.	Dysentery	462	78	258	0.17
6.	Accidents & Injuries	393	61	217	0.16
7.	Measles	54	355	214	6.57
8.	Gastro-enteritis	-	332	176	-
9.	Infantile liver	81	219	154	2.70
10.	Bronchitis	-	244	130	-

Sources : Office of the Registrar General—Survey on Infant and Child Mortality (1979)

MORBIDITY PATTERNS IN ANDHRA PRADESH

There are of course serious deficiencies in data as regards morbidity. Household surveys do not venture into the measurement of morbidity rates because the questions relating to sickness might not be properly asked and information elicited by non-medical investigators, especially from illiterate respondent. Thus, whatever data available with the public medical institutions, which maintain and process them are reported to the Ministry of Health and it publishes annually. Such data will not be useful to understand the health status of the people. Inspite of such serious limitation of the data, one could still make an attempt to know the broad trends and particularly the patterns of morbidity. We make one such attempt in this section.

Table 6 presents morbidity pattern from an all India survey of infant and child mortality. We have selected top nine sicknesses prevalent among infants (below one year) and presented them by sex. The most important disease among infants is septicaemia and pyaemia which is suffered by 4 per cent of infants. This disease is caused mainly by infection due to unhygienic surroundings and delivery practices at the home deliveries. The other diseases in the order of importance are tuberculosis, accidents and injuries, whooping cough and scabies. As the survey dates back in 1978, the preventable diseases through immunization are reported quite significantly. But now, the diseases may not be found in such a large scale. Again the gender bias exists in the incidence rates of the sicknesses. Septicaemia, whooping cough, and malaria is more than three times more prevalent among females than males.

Table 6 : Incidence rate of top nine sickness per 100,000 infants by sex in Urban Andhra Pradesh (1978)

S. No.	*Illness*	*Urban*			
		Male (M)	*Female (F)*	*Person (P)*	*F/M*
1.	Septicaemia and Pyaemia	180	600	403	3.33
2.	Tuberculosis of meanings and Central nervous system	374	403	389	1.08
3.	Accidents and Injuries	552	244	389	0.44
4.	Whooping Cough	156	541	360	3.47
5.	Scabies	298	406	355	1.36
6.	Malaria	54	173	118	3.20
7.	Poliomyelitis	-	219	116	-
8.	Diptheria	-	159	84	-
9.	Diseases of the circulatory system	69	-	53	-

Source : Office of the Registrar General—Survey on Infant the Child Mortality (1979)

Central Bureau of Health Intelligence (CBHI), Government of India publishes reported cases and deaths due to certain selected diseases. These data are based on the records of the public health institutions; and therefore do not reflect the morbidity rates as quite significant proportion of sicknesses are treated by private doctors, traditional medicine men and others. Also many diseases are not treated at all, because people consider them as not serious. Table 7 presents the reported cases and earths by selected diseases for all India and Andhra Pradesh during the calender year 1991. Cases as well as deaths in Andhra Pradesh, expressed as a percentage of All India are presented in the last column of the table. Nearly 16 per cent of all India diarrhoea cases are reported from Andhra Pradesh in 1991 and above 7 per cent deaths occurred in the state. Japan encephalitis is the second most prevalent diseases in Andhra Pradesh, with 13 per cent of cases and 14 per cent of death. In Andhra Pradesh meningitis constitute 11 per cent of all India cases, leprosy constitutes 10 per cent and S.T.D. 8 per cent of the cases.

Among communicable diseases, the most astonishing fact is that 43 per cent of cases of Diphtheria are reported from Andhra Pradesh, though the proportion of deaths due to the disease is 3. Tuberculosis constitutes nearly one-fourths of all India cases, whooping cough constitutes 145 per cent, enteric fever constitutes 13 per cent and Acute Respiratory Infection (ARI) constitutes 11 per cent of the total number of cases in India. If we look at the number of death due to the selected diseases, 18 per cent of all India deaths occurred due to ARI are reported from Andhra Pradesh. In Andhra Pradesh, Tuberculosis constitutes 13 per cent of total deaths and measles constitute about 11 per cent of deaths in India.

These data speaks volumes about the general performance of our immunization programme. Probably, the reported immunization coverage is either over reporting or untimely or incomplete. As child survival is the most important determinant of the successful family welfare programme, government should give top priority to the immunization programme.

Table 8 presents the number of deaths by major causes groups in All India and Andhra Pradesh during three years 1986, 1987 and 1988. Percentages of reported cases in Andhra Pradesh are calculated among all India cases and they are presented in the last columns of

Table 7 : Reported cases and deaths due to certain selected diseases in India and Andhra Pradesh (1991)

S. No.	Disease	All India Cases (C)	All India Deaths (D)	Case fatality Rate (D/C)	Andhra Pradesh Cases (C)	Andhra Pradesh Deaths (D)	Case fatality Rate (D/C)	Percentage of A.P. in All India Cases (C)	Percentage of A.P. in All India Deaths (D)
1.	Cholera	7088	150	2.12	119	2	1.68	1.68	1.33
2.	Diarrhoea	9280945	7493	0.08	1472821	551	0.04	15.87	7.35
3.	Malaria	2120472	421	0.02	82292	2	0.00	3.86	0.48
4.	Japan Encephalitis	3930	1482	37.71	528	213	40.34	13.44	14.37
5.	Meningitis	11995	2290	19.09	1333	59	4.43	11.11	2.58
6.	Leprosy[(1)]	2120020	-	-	214235	-	-	10.11	-
7.	S.T.D.[(2)]	1141740	-	-	86316	-	-	7.56	-
8.	*Communicable Diseases*								
	(a) Diptheria	12550	400	3.19	5340	11	0.21	42.55	2.75
	(b) Poliomyelitis	8670	181	2.09	726	1	0.14	8.37	0.55
	(c) Tetanus (Neo-natal)	11241	1101	9.79	304	19	6.25	2.70	1.73
	(d) Tetanus (Others)	15036	1872	12.45	752	136	18.09	5.01	7.26
	(e) Whooping Cough	73520	85	0.12	10603	7	0.07	14.42	8.24
	(f) Measles	79655	401	0.50	4436	42	0.95	5.57	10.47

(g) A.R.I.	10126044	3691	0.04	1145261	675	0.06	11.31	18.29
(h) Pneumonia	403337	3089	0.77	17940	71	0.40	4.45	2.30
(i) Enteric Fever	354143	1448	0.41	45326	46	0.10	12.80	3.18
(j) Tuberculosis	898047	8773	0.98	209565	1105	0.53	23.34	12.60

(1) Total number of cases recorded at the end of March 1991.

(2) Cases treated in STD clinics.

Source : Central Bureau of Health Intelligence—Health Information of India (1992).

Table 8 : Number of deaths by major cause groups in All India and Andhra Pradesh (1986-88)

S. No.	*Cause of Death*	*All India*			*Andhra Pradesh*			*Percentage of A.P. in All India*		
		1986	*1987*	*1988*	*1986*	*1987*	*1988*	*1986*	*1987*	*1988*
1.	Accidents and Injuries	1269	1311	1489	104	120	96	8.20	9.15	6.45
2.	Child Birth and Pregnancies	176	197	182	17	8	4	9.66	4.06	2.20
3.	Fevers	1894	1898	1819	84	66	92	4.44	3.48	5.06
4.	Digestive disorders	1410	1459	1497	110	112	92	7.80	7.68	6.15
5.	Coughs (Disorders of respiratory systems)	3606	4053	4657	163	232	182	4.52	5.72	3.91
6.	Disorders of the Central nervous system	684	793	1059	96	72	99	14.04	9.08	9.35
7.	Disorders of circulatory system	1649	1935	2304	107	114	108	6.49	5.89	4.69
8.	Other clear symptoms	1561	1880	2020	129	144	149	8.26	7.66	7.38
9.	Causes peculiar to infancy	1923	2056	2256	150	145	153	7.80	7.05	6.78
10.	Senility	4090	4659	5667	403	418	435	9.85	8.97	7.68
	Total	18262	20241	22950	1363	1431	1410	7.46	7.07	6.14

Source : Central Bureau of Health Intelligence (CBHI)—Health Information in India (1992).

the table. Percentage of deaths in Andhra Pradesh among all India has fallen from 7.5 per cent in 1986 to 6.1 per cent in 1988. There is a significant decrease in the proportion of deaths due to problems related to child birth and pregnancies in Andhra Pradesh (10 per cent in 1986 to 2 per cent in 1988). On the other hand there is a marginal increase in the percentage of deaths due to fever (4 per cent in 1986 to 5 per cent in 1988). Overall, the proportions of all the diseases in Andhra Pradesh are reported to be decreasing during the three year period.

Table 9 presents reported number of cases of Cholera, Diarrhoea diseases, Malaria, Japanese Encephalitis, Meningitis and Leprosy in Andhra Pradesh and All India during the years of 1990, 1991 and 1992. Surprisingly, more than one fifths of all the cases of Meningitis in India are reported in A.P. in 1992. This proportion has been increasing over time. In 1990, there were only 9%, and this increased to 11% in 1991. Next highest incidence of the disease reported in A.P. is diarrhoea with 16% of all the cases in India in 1991. The third major disease prevalent in A.P. is leprosy. About 16% of all the new cases in India are reported in A.P. during 1991-92. Though, Japan encephalitis is reported to have declined in 1991, the proportion of cases reported was 23% in 1990.

CONCLUSIONS AND POLICY IMPLICATIONS

Andhra Pradesh is poised for a situation of lower mortality and higher morbidity, posing a challenge to the government which is already facing acute shortage of resources for investing in the health sector. Although, general mortality rates are declining, still there are alarmingly higher perinatal and neo-natal mortality rates. Surprisingly, still birth rate is higher in urban areas than in rural areas. Urban infant mortality rate in Andhra Pradesh has been on the increase during most part of the past decade 1981-1991. Prevalence of certain diseases like ARI and Diptheria are alarmingly high in the state, which requires immediate attention of the Government.

The above empirical evidence demonstrates that there is something wrong with the health status of urban population in Andhra Pradesh understandably, does not improve with the increase in the number of medical and health institutions because health is a function not only of medical care but of the overall integrated development of society—social, economic and cultural. The objectives of integrated development are to eliminate poverty and inequality, to spread

Table 9 : Reported cases of certain selected diseases in A.P. & All India (1990-1992).

	A.P.				All India	
	Cases	*% in All India*	*Deaths*	*% in All India*	*Cases*	*Deaths*
1. Reported Cases & deaths due to Cholera & Diarrhoeal Diseases :						
1990 : Cholera	69	1.86	0	(0)	3704	87
Diarrhoea	1086233	11.34	424	4.91	9579738	8633
1991 : Cholera	119	1.68	2	1.33	7088	150
Diarrhoea	1472821	15.87	551	7.35	9280945	7493
2. Positive Cases of Malaria & Deaths :						
1990	104483	5.18	5	1.42	2018783	353
1991	82292	3.88	2	0.48	2120472	421
3. Reported cases of Japanese Encephalitis :						
1990	667	22.87	293	22.70	2916	1291
1991	528	13.44	213	14.37	3930	1482
4. Reported Cases of Meningitis :						
1990	1516	9.05	75	2.51	16757	2984

1991	1333	11.11	59	2.58	11995	2290
1992	1872	20.68	40	2.37	9051	1685
5. Recorded Prevalence Rate of Leprosy (1991-92) :						
Total No. of Cases recorded at the end of March 1991 :	2,14,235	10.11			21,20,020	-
New Cases 1991-92 :	80,007	15.60			5,12,836	-

Source : Central Bureau of Health Intelligence—Health Information of India (1992).

education and to enable the poor and underprivileged to assert themselves. Health development can be integrated with larger programme of overall development in such a manner that the two become mutually self supporting.

Urban society is a highly heterogeneous group with higher the size of the population, higher will be the inequalities in housing environment and other living conditions. The slum population is a 'floating' migratory group that is both economically and socially deprived. Coupled with the non-availability of health services and poor living conditions it is a fact that this group has no traditional system of health care to fall back upon. This group is under greater risk of growing incidence of STD and HIV cases, which require greater awareness among people regarding safer sexual practices coupled with backup medical and health services, which are easily acceptable and affordable. Government do not seem to be focusing much on reproductive health as they do for family planning or immunization. Still birth rate, peri-natal and neo-natal mortality rates are very much linked with the availability of reproductive health care services apart from nutritional status, age at conception, educational status of the mother and a host of other social and cultural factors. Therefore, it is strongly recommended that the socio-economic development programmes in the urban areas should not be neglected and health education programmes should be stepped up together with backup reproductive health care services to the urban poor.

REFERENCES

1. Johansson R.S. - 1991, "The Health Transition : the Cultural Inflation of Morbidity during the Decline of Mortality" *Health Transition Review,* Vol. 1, No. 1.
2. Gopalakrishna Kumar - 1993, "Low Mortality and High Morbidity in Kerala Reconsidered" *Population Development Review,* Vol. 19, No. 1, March 1993.
3. Rao B.S., and Ramachandrudu G. - 1991, "Report on the Household Survey" Evaluation Study of the Visakhapatnam Slum Improvement Project, IDPS, (mimeo).
4. Registrar General, India, - 1991, Sample Registration System, "Fertility and Mortality Indicators".
5. Ministry of Health and Family Welfare, "Family Welfare Year Book 1990-91".

6. Central Bureau of Health Intelligence (CBHI), - 1992, "Health Information in India".
7. Caldwell J.C., - 1989 "Introductory Thoughts on Health Transition" in Caldwell, et. al, (1989) "What do we know about Health Transition?" Australian National University, Canberra.
8. Jain A.K. and Judith Bruce, - 1993, "Implications of Reproductive Health for Objectives and Efficiency of Family Planning Programme". The Population Council Working paper, No. 8.
9. Office of the Registrar General, - 1979, "Survey on Infant and Child Mortality.

SECTION C

SOCIAL ASPECTS OF HEALTH STATUS

9

SOCIO-CULTURAL DETERMINANTS OF HEALTH STATUS OF RURAL WOMEN

Dr. P. Durga Prasad

INTRODUCTION

Wholesome fulfilment of the national goals of overall social and economic development requires, among other things, provision of health and family welfare services through a mechanism which not only makes these services available but ensures that they are accessible, affordable and appropriate.

The recommendations of the committee on "Health Survey and Development (Bhore Committee, 1946)" laid the foundation for the present form of organisation and delivery of health services in the country through the primary health care approach. Beginning with the community development programmes of 1952 and with the impetus provided by a variety of planned programmes through the successive Five-Year Plans, health care in India seems to have made significant strides in terms of decreased mortality rates, increased life expectancy at birth, better nutrition and sanitation on the one hand, and improved infrastructure, higher allocation of financial, material and manpower resources on the other. However, owing both to the problems of a rapidly growing population and an erosion in the resource base and the quality of health services, there appears a serious gap in the management of health care, notably in rural areas as is reflected, for example, by the following :

(i) Mortality rates of women and children continue to be high. Nearly a third of the total deaths occur in children below the age of 5 years. Infant mortality was reported at about 95 per thousand in 1985 at the national level. However, across the states this figure varies. U.P. has a high 147, Gujarat recorded 111 and Kerala accounted for the lowest at 30. Maternal mortality rate was nearly 4 per thousand.

(ii) Malnutrition continues to affect expectant and lactating mothers and children adversely. About 50 per cent of women in general and about 70 per cent during pregnancy suffer as a result of malnutrition. Protein-calorie and other nutritional deficiencies are extremely high among children. Over 27 million children are at risk each year.

(iii) In 1981, over a third of the Indian villages were declared 'problematic' areas for potable water. Only 2 per cent of the rural population has good sanitation facilities.

(vi) The performance of the Family Planning Programme has not been satisfactory. The birth rate continues to be high at 33 per thousand.

(v) Less than two-thirds of infants and expectant mothers are covered against the six vaccine-preventable diseases through the programme of immunization.

(vi) Problems of leprosy face four million people.

(vii) Over 10 million persons suffer from TB.

(viii) There are nine million blind persons. About 45 million suffer from visual impairment.

(ix) A variety of diseases such as malaria, filaria, goitre, vitamin deficiency problems, worm infestations, skin infections and other health problems continue to cause disability, panic and death among million.*

Towards closing the gaps as above, the government has rededicated itself to achieving the desired standards of health both by way of overhauling the existing health system and more importantly, by subscribing rigorously to the Alma-Ata philosophy of primary health care approach to health, rural health in particular. Such an exercise in overhauling the existing health system requires not only provision/re-organisation of various inputs and services but also a thorough

---

* Data for items (i) to (ix) are based on figures provided in the statistical volume "Health Information of India, 1987" DGHS, Ministry of Health and Family Welfare, GOI, New Delhi, 1987.

understanding of the non-medical factors—socio-cultural factors in other words, that affect the health status of women, rural women in particular. Health in India involves the interplay of several socio-cultural factors. However, the damaging role played by the socio-cultural milieu in problems of health and disease does not attract the kind of attention it deserves. The paper endeavours to present an analysis of these factors as also spell out implications for the well-being of women—women, who, for a variety of social and other reasons did not get to enjoy equal and free access to health.

The Influence of Ritual Practices on Health

That 'the performance of rituals is intimately connected with religious beliefs in Indian culture' is a familiar theme to many of us. Beliefs about the relationship of human beings to the supernatural forces in the Universe are legion. Sickness in Indian villages, by and large, signifies moral as well as a physical crisis, involving human conduct as cosmic purpose. Those women suffering from physical weakness owing to anaemia, etc., are given/ought to be given strength restoring inputs like balanced diets coupled with iron and folic acid tablets and vitamins, if their problem is visualised from the perspective of modern allopatic medicine. However, the ritual (Hindu) cure for the same prescribes a ritual pilgrimage that envisages ritual baths/holy dips in Ganges, Yamuna, Godavari, for example. This year, the Ganges (Kumbh Mela) witnessed the pouring in of lakhs of human beings into its waters for ritual baths.

Dhillon, et al (1965) found that, to a great extent the Malaria spraying campaigns in Orissa did not succeed due to the cultural practice of frequent plastering of both inner and outer house walls. On average, 8-10 plasterings a year were done either to celebrate festivals or to remove pollution after childbirth or as part of preparations for marriage.

In Maharashtra, Gujarat and Rajasthan puberty, virginity and fertility related rituals galore. Young women are perforce made to undertake ritual trips to places (e.g. villages near Mt. Abu) believed to be known for either conferring benefits/boons on them or removing the evils relating to the above instead of a proper treatment of such critical/sensitive problems. The consequences can well be imagined.

In villages of Andhra Pradesh, Gujarat and West Bengal (perhaps true of many other places), ritual occupies a pride of place in being visualised as 'medicine' for 'healing' the 'sick'. Rituals that include worship of goddesses Mysamma, Mariamma, Chinna Ammavaru, Pedda Ammavaru (Choti/Bari Mata), Sitala, Celaibibi abound. Apart from serving the objectives of individual well-being, some of these rituals are reportedly performed for the community well-being too.

Akhtar (1977) notes that apart from dietetic variations among the Hindus and Muslims, certain other cultural rituals affect health. Uterine cancer amongst Hindu women was twice higher than that of Muslim women in spite of their (Muslim women) early marriage and a higher number of pregnancies. This major difference between the two religious communities, the author believes, may be attributed to the fact that Muslim males are circumcised in accordance with the Islamic ritual. And circumcision, as is widely believed and scientifically founded, has perhaps been an aid to lowering the incidence of Uterine cancer. Like-wise, Paymaster (1964) also records that the incidence of cervix cancer was higher amongst the sample Hindu women of Bombay.

To sum up, the 'rituals' illustrated testify that people believe that 'little can be done by themselves to restore health' and, hence, accord higher priority, on the scale of their values, to those ceremonies and practices that purport to maintain harmony between themselves and their supernatural world.

Beliefs, Customs, Traditions and Supersititions

Beliefs relating to illness tend to inhibit the acceptance of etiological and other causes of disease, and treatment of the same, therefore, becomes more difficult. Perceptions about the link between food habits and disease are aplenty. The belief that certain foods are "heat producing" while the others are "cold producing", pervades all over the countryside. Nations as regards which kinds (as above) of foods are to be taken, and when (season) and in what combination are also quite widespread as also vary considerably geographically. Foods believed to produce 'heat' in the North are considered 'cold' producing in the South. Whatever be the differences in the range of foods and their combinations across geographical regions, the belief that "failure to follow the eating rules of the game" would inevitably result in the occurrence of malfunctions in the body is widely shared all over.

Hassan (1967) reports from his study of a village in Lucknow that the villagers think that it is the quantity of food eaten that matters for the health of a person. The idea of quantity of food is often left out from their realm of thinking.

It is in the above context as also that of the foregoing that the status of health of several rural women is adversely affected, for prescriptions and proscriptions are applied more rigorously in the case of women than the others. The incidence of malnutrition is considerably high amongst both the expectant and nursing mothers. Country-wide, about 50 per cent of women in general and about 70 per cent during pregnancy suffer as a result of malnutrition. The material mortality rate was 4 per thousand, as already pointed out.

Field observations also reveal that certain diseases may be attributable to the food choices. The high incidence of stomach cancer in the South may be due to the excessive consumption of fats and chillies while in Gujarat contrastingly, where less pungent foods are taken together with dairy products, the incidence of cancer of the stomach is lower.

Cancers of mouth and lips are common in many of those pats of the country where consumption of pan and tobacco (smoke as well as in raw form) in prevalent. Those rural women, the agricultural and other labourers in particular in Gujarat and A.P. addicted to smoking cigarettes and beedies, may suffer most from problems of lip and mouth cancer. Some women of Srikakulám and Guntur districts of A.P. are known for reverse smoking, which causes lip cancer.

PROHIBITED FOODS

In all cultures the staple food is cooked and eaten according to certain rules, manners, customs and traditions, and rites and taboos prevalent in the society. The taboos, prejudices, beliefs and attitudes centering around food are also products of cultural practices that are in vogue. These are known to block full utilization of available food, and thus create and/or aggravate malnutrition. Elimination of certain foods from the dietary basket may be attributed to the practice of certain customs and prejudices. Thus 'Ragi' in Karnataka and 'Bajra' in Maharashtra that are considered staple foods are frowned upon in parts of UP and Gujarat. The Christians consider pork a delicacy but to a Muslim eating the same is short of blasphemy. Thus, some pregnant women recommended consumption of Ragi in Mangalore district by the Health Workers, did not take it kindly, for Ragi was considered a 'poor man's' food. Consequently, a potential gain in their calorie-intake could not materialise. Similarly, consumption of wheat (Roti or bread) in the coastal districts of A.P. is kept at bare minimum or not consumed at all, for roti/bread are visualised as 'patient (sickness) foods'.

Age and sex selective food restriction related to food habits are not uncommon. Such groups, by and large, include expectant and lactating mothers, and widows. In fact, it is common place to find that food linked prejudices are interested with the religio-cultural beliefs specific to each of the social groups.

Apte (1977) notes from his field observations in Tamil Nadu that low income people believe that soda water cures many ills in pregnancy, so they buy it instead of nutritious food available for the same amount of money. They also believed that consumption of leafy vegetables by pregnant women will lead to the birth of dark skinned babies. Leftover foods are avoided by lactating mothers, so that a women who can not afford to cook at fresh meal for herself in the morning has to do without any food.

The author's field observations in MP and Gujarat reveal that pregnant women of Sihore, and Bhavnagar districts shun consumption of eggs (a rich cheap and easily available source of protein) as they believed that eating of eggs will result in the birth of bald babies. Similarly, certain foods are prescribed during puberty, menstruation, pregnancy and lactation stages. For example, in Gujarat, papaya is anathema to many Gujaratis in general and females (young and pregnant) in particular so much so that papaya is not even grown domestically—it is totally tabooed. Many varieties of vegetarian and particularly non-vegetarian foods are avoided as they are believed to transmit diseases to children through the mother's breast milk.

SOCIAL STATUS, LIFE-STYLES AND THEIR IMPACT

Both the quality and quantity, and the variety of food intake often assumes one of the major expressions of wealth and status in the Indian Communities. The reference group theory (in the sense of having some models for emulation or sanskritization in other words) seems to explain a part of the behaviour of people in this context. Most people would often like to depict behaviour that is in line with 'what they want to be' rather than express 'what they are'. For example, in some parts of Karnataka, Ragi, once considered poor man's food came to be viewed as desirable because the Maharaja of Waudier ate Ragi at every meal.

Highlighting the problem of malnutrition in South India, Rao (1962) observed that there is no concept of deficiency diseases, but foods are graded by their prestige value. Poor people with little money may begin (the author observed this actually happening) to compromise on buying a few drops of groundnut oil at a high cost rather than go for palm oil that is less expensive because groundnut oil is consumed by the higher income families. Similar is the case of choice between sugar and gur (unrefined sugar) or milk (animal) protein and soya (vegetable) protein wherein sugar and milk win over due to considerations of class, prestige, etc., though gur and soya are less expensive as also more nutritious per unit of consumption. Such tendencies may be harmful to women, particularly the poor and pregnant/lactating mothers, for they might well be foregoing major energy giving/money saving inputs to health in favour of the intangible and unproductive notions of class and prestige.

Cultural notions of work land their effect on hygiene and sanitation. Beginning with the hygiene and sanitation programmes of the community development programmes, a large number of such programmes have been on but with little impact. One of the major reasons for the relatively low subscription of people to such concept as domestic or community hygiene, and sanitation is said to be related to the cultural notions of people/social groups. The Community Compost Pits Programme, for example, did not catch up in several places of Gujarat mainly due to the high-clean caste cultural notions of work that "only low-caste people or servants should/can carry the domestic refuse out through the streets into the community compost pit". Thus, the sanitation programme suffered serious setbacks even before the turn of the week it was introduced. Unhygienic conditions surely can affect both males and females equally. However, women particularly pregnant/lactating mothers perhaps suffer more than the men, for women are more susceptible to catching air/fly borne diseases during such critical times. The consequences could be quite serious.

SUMMARY AND CONCLUSIONS

The cherished goal of all planned efforts is to ensure well-being of the people through supportive and developmental programmes. Health care in rural areas and of women in particular is one such major developmental programme and, hence, deserves high priority in both research and investment terms.

It is well known that human behaviour is largely a product of the socio-cultural milieu into which human beings are socialized. Analysts have established beyond doubt that the success of any development programme largely depends on behaviour. Health is no exception to this.

Field studies on rural social, political, economic and cultural life are now widely available. However, field studies on the intimate relationship between rural socio-cultural factors and health have been few and far between. Consequently, there is little knowledge about the beliefs, customs, rituals, traditions, taboos and practices of rural people in so far as their health and disease are concerned and particularly the manner in which their life ways affect their health status. It is perhaps for this reason that the public health authorities are unable to encourage the people to increasingly utilize their services, for necessary knowledge of the relationship between the two broad phenomena as above, is either deficient or altogether lacking amongst the health promoters. There is thus an urgent need to understand the socio-cultural context in which health workers have to relate to the people so as to make meaningful and sustained interventions.

One of the communal aspects of village is the existence of a common set of standards, beliefs, values and norms of behaviour which are referred to by individuals deciding whether or not to adopt health practices. Since people need support for their actions, often they tend to conform to the standard behaviour of the majority members of the community. Hence, if they do not do so, they think their social relationships and social values get affected. These are often ignored by outsiders coming in contact with villagers who assume that their programme aims and means are convergent with those of the people. Local beliefs form a coherent system which provide explanations for events otherwise beyond the scientific comprehension of many societies. Sometimes the rationale behind certain beliefs is apparent : for e.g., diets of pregnant women are said to be restricted because people believe that this will ensure a small baby and easy delivery. Other beliefs such as ritual pollution of upper caste members by the other caste members are less easy to comprehend. What is fundamental, however, is that beliefs relating whether to religion, health, food or any such activity, are all interrelated to form a closed system with which failures can be explained. Thus, the failure of folk medicine is accepted because the patient was beyond help whereas the failure of a doctor to treat and cure a symptom is not easily accepted.

To ensure that one initiates the right course of action in rural health programmes, it would be instructive to keep the foregoing socio-cultural factors in mind. The interventionists would do well if they could attempt to eliminate the negative influences of those factors as also make use of the positive ones.

REFERENCES

1. Akthar, R. and A. Learmonth, "The Resurgence of Malaria in India: 1965-76", Geo-Journal, Vol. 1, No. 5, 1977, p. 71.
2. Apte, J.K., "The Social Cultural Aspects of Food Avoidance in a Low Income Population" in Tamil Nadu, Journal of Tropical Paediatrics, Environment and Child Health, Vol. 23, No. 2, 1977, pp. 83-90.
3. Dhillon, H.S. and S.B. Kar, "Malaria Eradication and Investigation of Cultural Patterns and Beliefs among Tribal Population in India", International Journal of Health Education, Vol. III, No. 1, 1965, pp. 31-40.
4. Hassan, K.A., Cultural Frontiers of Health in Village India, Bombay, 1967.
5. Paymaster, T.C., "Cancer and its Distribution in India", Cancer, Vol. 17, 1964, pp. 1026-34.
6. Rao, K.S., "Malnutrition in South India", in A. Bargers and R.F.A. Dean (eds.) Malnutrition and Food Habits, London, 1962.

10

HEALTH PROBLEMS OF THE SLUM DWELLER IN THE CITY OF VISAKHAPATNAM

Dr. K. Sreeranjani Subba Rao, Ph. D.

The aim of the paper is to focus on the health hazards faced by the slum dwellers or the Urban poor in the area of Visakhapatnam Municipal Corporation.

Visakhapatnam is one of the fast growing cities of Asia. It is growing rapidly due to the industries like Steel Plant, Port, Caltex, Coromandel, Bharat Heavy Plates and Vessels Limited and other educational and medical institutions. The rapid growth of the city is causing a number of changes. Since more and more people from the surrounding villages are flocking around to the city in search of jobs for their living, they fall to find enough the proper accommodation. As the rental values of the houses are very high a large number of migrated people are constructing hutments which is gradually growing towards a slum area. This is how slums are coming up in the city. In Visakhapatnam, there are 170 slums areas with a total population of 2 lakhs, out of 8 lakhs of the total population of Visakhapatnam, The migrated unemployed population who lives in the slum areas are mostly low wage income earners working in different industries.

The dwellers of the slums being predominantly poor are facing a number of problems which they arc very common like housing, water, drainage, sanitary along with health problems which are very common in the slum areas. So far no systematic studies have been made on the health standards of the slum dwellers of the city of Visakhapatnam. Hence the present paper is an attempt to project some of the health problems faced by the Urban poor in the city of Visakhapatnam.

As most of the slums are located on the banks of some drains without having the minimum civic rights like drainage, drinking water, lighting, toilets, roads, pathways etc., they become the tools of the disease dispersals. Due to the unhygienic surroundings of the slum areas become areas of fastly spreading diseases. The poverty will add as a catalyst due to their malnutrition and hence the diseases will spread as epidemics so much that the health hazards become a challenging problems.

Poverty, ignorance and disease i.e., the (triangle triad) one leading to the basic problem with regard to the healthy condition of the slum dwellers. Though there are major Govt. Hospitals like King George Hospital, Govt. Victoria Hospital for women and children, Rani Candramani Devi Hospital, Tuberclosis and Infectious diseases Hospital, and E.S.I. which are catering services to many people—the slum dwellers very often approach the Quacks (Unqualified doctors) or radical shops to get primary treatment and temporary relief. This inadequate treatment leads to chronic diseases that keeps them out of their jobs resulting shattering of the family. Majority of the slum dwellers expressed their transport problems since most of the slum areas are far away from the big Govt. Hospitals. Hence the slum dwellers even today for any immunization are going to the private doctors.

Another treating problem is the maternity and child care. The pregnant mothers are quite ignorant about the care to be taken during pregnancy and child birth, delivery and post delivery, unhygienic methods leading to infectious diseases resulting in abortions and miscarriages which finally causes ill health to the mother. Here the Dais (Untrained midwives) are responsible for making the delivery more complicated by following the unscientific methods during the time of delivery. The neonatal and post-natal children do not have any facility for their normal growth as the mothers are illiterates. Due to the illiteracy and ignorance the slum dwellers do not know anything about the immunization programme to the children which is absolutely necessary in the first year of child birth. The mal-nutrition adds to the problem producing unhealthy child which becomes another challenge to the corporation. Children are not able to be looked after by their labour parents who are busy in earning money for their livelihood.

The next health-striken people are Gereatric group consisting above 60 years. These aged people are not taken by this working class due to poverty and are not given proper nourishment leading to ill-health. This group is called the Vulnerable group.

With a view to provide overall improvement the Visakhapatnam Municipal Corporation has been taking up a number of rehabilitation programmes.

(1) One of its main aim is to make a comprehensive study of the common diseases of the slum dwellers.

(2) Free clinics have been established in the slum areas. The aim of these free clinics is not only to attend immediate medical care but also to promote health and to prevent diseases.

(3) In order to promote medical facilities to the door steps of the slum areas, the VMC has planned to select one person from each slum area and train him to identify their medical problems so that the Corporation could take necessary steps.

(4) To provide immediate care to the pregnant women the VMC is constructing community labour rooms where immediate care will be given to the pregnant women at the time of delivery. If the case is serious, they will direct the patient to go to major Hospitals like King George Hospital or Victoria Government Hospital.

Some suggestions to improve the health conditions of the slum dwellers

(1) To give training to the youth and women in the slum areas to take leadership so that they can think about their problems and possible solutions.

(2) To create welfare centres for women and train the women in traditional handicrafts so that they can earn their bread. This also helps the women to pay more attention on their children as they need not go out for earning.

(3) To shoulder the responsibility for their own development voluntary organisations should make deliberate attempts by preaching the evils of alcoholism and smoking and other drug addicts.

(4) To make the slum dwellers to realise the importance of the population proverb, "Health is Wealth", and that this has a pivotal role for the betterment of their entire family.

I am thankful to the Municipal authorities for giving me the necessary data in the preparation of this paper. I also express my sincere thanks to Dr. B. Swaraja Lakshmi, Retd. Prof. of Social and Preventive Medicine, Andhra Medical College, Visakhapatnam for her suggestions and encouragement.

11

HEALTH FOR ALL BY 2000 A.D. — NEED FOR SOCIAL CHANGE

Prof. G. Parthasarathy

I seek to answer three questions in this note. They are :

(1) What do the empirical data on impact indicators of health convey on the progress of health since the Alma Ata conference in 1978?

(2) What are the lessons of the Direct Intervention Programme under primary health care, mainly ICDS, and what are the directions in which such direct interventions need to be strengthened?

(3) What are the relative roles of state and society in contributing to the goal of health for all by 2000 A.D., and what are the policy directions ?

A critical impact indicator of health is infant mortality. I look at the infant mortality rates presented by my friend Prof. S. Chandrasekhar in his recent instructive book, "Towards 2000 A.D. Indian Health Economy and Policy". The data convey three messages.

(a) Infant mortality declined in Andhra Pradesh since the late 1970s. This is gratifying. For Andhra Pradesh, as a whole, the rate declined from around 120 per 1,000 in 1976 to less than 80 in the late 1980s. Such decline is noticeable for both urban and rural areas.

(b) The rates of infant mortalities continue to be higher for rural areas, urban slums, for landless labour, for scheduled caste, scheduled tribes and for rural muslim population, as compared to Hindu and Christian, population.

As in 1985, rural infant mortality rates in Andhra Pradesh are one-and-half times the corresponding infant mortality rate for urban areas. Rural muslim infant mortality rates, as seen from recorded, data were 1.18 times the infant mortalities for rural Hindus. Rural scheduled caste infant mortality rates in Andhra Pradesh are 1.12 times and of rural schedules tribe infant mortality rates are 1.22 times. Socially and economically backward and poorer groups in society and rural areas continue to show higher health risks. These are also the groups which record lower levels of literacy, nutrition and higher incidence of poverty.

(c) A third important message of the data relates to the status of woman, and progress in health. In households with illiterate women both in rural and urban areas, infant mortality rates are much higher; more than one-and-half times the corresponding rates for households with literate women. Worker participation among women, and consequently relatively more independent status also contributes to decline in infant mortality rates. Even more telling is the age at marriage of women. For women married at less than the age of 18, infant mortality rates in rural Andhra Pradesh were double the corresponding infant mortality rates for women married at 18 and above.

A fourth important message is that the *rates of decline* in infant mortality slowed down in the 80s compared to 70s as health programmes had to reckon with social groups which were more prone to health risks. This suggests that the tasks in the decade 90s are going to the more challenging than the earlier decade.

The policy shift to Primary Health Care has been fruitful and it has been found to reduce the health risks. An important component of the Primary Health Care system is the Integrated Child Development Service, familiarly known as ICDS. Effective and improved functioning of the ICDS is critical for meeting the challenges of the decade 1990s. A friend of mine Prof. K. Subba Rao prepared a discussion paper, entitled "Improving Nutrition in India", for the World Bank in 1989. He evaluated the impact of ICDS Project Reports released by the Monitoring Cell and available on a continuous basis for years 1978, 1979, 1982-84, and 1984-85. The projects were evaluated in terms of their impact on the status of malnourished children (less than 60% weight for age). The conclusion of this carefully conducted study are useful. Definite improvement was perceptable only in 25 per cent of the projects in rural areas, and 60 per cent of the projects in urban areas. These findings of poor nutritional impact in a significant number of projects are also supported by the findings of the National Institute of Public Cooperation in Child Development. The most important deficiency in the functioning of ICSSR is noted to be the low average of children under three years of age and even lower coverage of pregnant and lactating women. A study in Medak district in Andhra Pradesh, 1985 showed that nearly a half of the infant deaths could have been prevented by immunisation and oral rehydration therapy. Clearly, if ORT and immunisation were systematically practised in the Anganwadi the mortality rate could have fallen. The neglect of 0-3 children was noted even in relation to supplementary feeding in another study in Gujarat and Maharashtra. Further food supplied to ICDS centres were found to be erratic. Another deficiency noted in the study of Nutrition Foundation of India in 1988 is the weak link of ICDS with the health infrastructure. The number of medical officers, Lady Health visitors, auxiliary nurses and midwives fall behind the sanctioned strength in many states. Quality of training also needed improvement, further, there has been a need for converting the prevailing status of ICDS from 'Government centres' into 'Community centres'.

The most popular view best articulated in the National Foundation of Nutrition Study is that ICDS is a well-conceived programme reflecting a bold and innovative approach; many of its observed ills can be removed by effective implementation. Its observed deficiencies could be corrected. These are : (a) the relative failure to reach the children below 3 years and pregnant and lactating women, (b) the poor health and nutrition education, and (c) the neglect of home visits and community participation. The World Bank discussion paper suggests two women workers for Anganwadi, one for pre-school, and another to look after infants and pregnant women, nutritional education and home visits, as an experimental measure. This suggestion needs to be considered for better functioning of ICDS.

As regards the role of the state the National Front Government has expressed its deep commitment to a more widely diffused growth and concentration of public investment in areas with high concentration of poverty. This should help in accelerating the development of health and related social infrastructure, particularly drinking water supply and primary education in rural areas. The focus on the local decentralised development should help in the choice of critical location specific health infrastructure. However, the utilisation of such access by poorer groups, most prone to health risks, depends upon the improvement in employment and incomes progress in poverty alleviation and their impowerment within the rural areas.

I will only dwell on a couple of aspects in which society, particularly the elite leadership has a role. It is in the health field, that ethics and self-interest converge. It is ethical to be concerned with the health of fellow human beings. It is also in the self-interest of the elite group since health of a poor man has externalities which affect the whole community. But there are unhealthy and growing trends of individualism, privatisation, competitive acquisition and consumerism cutting at the root of the ethical base of society. In my view the elite in society has a role in reversing these trends, not by mere professions but by effective demonstration in their lives.

Secondly, nothing is more critical to the progress in health than the status of women, her level of education, her participation in the decision making of the household, and the age at what she is married.

'Health for all by 2000 A.D.' to be translated into a reality, should be backed up by strong social movements for improving the status of women in the society. Societies change only slowly. But young with vision dedication and commitment, could accelerate the change. Let me hope that 'Health for all' will be a reality.

12

HEALTH TRANSITION AND THE ROLE OF LITERACY

Prof. (Mrs.) K. Ranigopal

INTRODUCTION

The issue of health of great importance both from the point of view of the individuals and the nation as well. In any country it is the health status of the people that determine the pace of economic development and the well-being of the people Health is an important problem both in the advanced and developing countries. However, it is a serious problem in the developing countries. Health status of the people determines the average expectation of life, number of people in productive age bracket, production productivity, earning capacity, employment and welfare of the people. On the other hand several economic variables like income, employment, purchasing power, quality and quantity of goods and services available etc. determine the health status of the people.

It is a widely recognised fact that human capital plays dominant role in the context of economic development, as it accounts for major portion of the growth of an economy. Health is an important component of human capital. There is indeed a vicious circle present in the developing countries like India which is as follows :

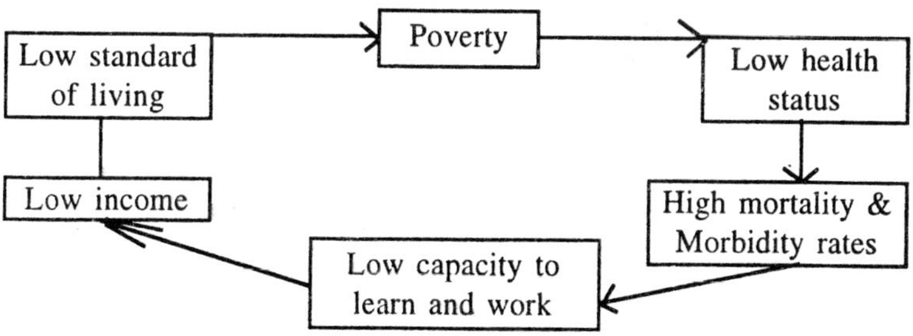

This vicious circle needs to be broke in the interests of the growth of the economy and promotion of the welfare of the people. It may be done through enhancing the health status of the people, as it will go a long way in eliminating wastage of human resources i.e. in terms of mortality, morbidity, disability and debility. Indeed health status exercises profound influence on human resource development and effective utilisation of human resources.

In 1978 at the international conference on primary health care, the health Assembly of WHO, in Alma Ata, it was unanimously decided that primary health care on all is essential and it is an integral part of social development in the spirit of special equity and justice. India is also a signatory to the Resolution and is committed to the attainment of the goal of health for all by 2000 AD through Universal provision of comprehensive primary health care services. The concept of primary health care implies access for all to minimum health care close to their homes to enable every citizen to lead a healthy economically productive and socially satisfying life.

Health Transition

Against this background it is highly essential to find out the changes in the health status of the people from time to time as it helps in taking right steps so as to achieve or go nearer to the goal of health for all by 2000 AD. Moreover periodical assessment of the change in the health status of the people is necessary to bring about suitable changes in the policy and approach depending on the changed conditions needs and problems of the society and health sector. In India mortality has come down but morbidity is still high and that led to low health status of the people. It implies nothing but prolonging the lives of those in the substandard state of health. Health care and medical facilities programmes initiated and executed since the advent of planning have been helpful in bringing down the death rate and incidence of communicable diseases. Expectation of life has increased. Approximately five fold increase in the number of hospital beds accompanied by an increase of around 150 per cent in the number of hospitals and dispensaries bear testimony to the improvement in the health infrastructure. The rapid increase in the number of medical colleges and enrolment in them ensures the feasibility of continued improvements on the health care front.

Mortality has come down considerably after 1921 and particularly after independence. But there is no significant fall in the incidence of sickness. In this connection it is worth pointing out that reliable time series data regarding morbidity is not available. It may be pointed out that India has moved from the first phase of high mortality and morbidity into the second phase of health transition i.e. of lower mortality but still high morbidity.

Rural-Urban Differences : One of the main reasons for the poor state of health of the people is wrong priorities as far as resource allocation is concerned. There has been a progressive reduction in budgetary allocation for health in successive five year plans. Only Rs. 3 per head per mensum is spent on health. Moreover these meagre resources are unevenly distributed. Nearly 80 per cent is spent on big hospitals in metropolitan cities and large urban areas, which cater to less than 20 per cent of the population whereas 20 per cent of resources are spent on primary health care which caters to 80 per cent of the people.

About 525 million people (76.6%) live in rural areas (1981 census) having inadequate health and medical care facilities. This large population is scattered over 5.76 lakhs villages. Only 30 per cent of the rural people are able to read and write. Poverty prevails widely in the countryside. Using calorie consumption as criterion 37 per cent of the total population live below the poverty line. Moreover in rural areas people do not have proper water, housing and sanitation facilities. With low incomes, high level of illiteracy and strong ethnic and linguistic bonds it has been a challenge to the central and state governments to improve the level of living of the rural people .

Although during the early post independence period the emphasis was more on the provision of increased medical care facilities of the Government realised the need to pay equal attention to preventive, promotive and public health aspects of health care. The shift in emphasis has been evolved over successive five year plans. Development of health services in India through primary health care approach started with the recommendation and guidance provided by the health survey and development committee (Bhore committee) in 1946. To meet the comprehensive health needs of the population primary health centres were set up throughout the country after considerable thought. Their functioning and coverage are still inadequate and the situation is paradoxical with changing needs and a static system of health care.

Our country is divided into 22 major states and 9 smaller union territories and 431 districts. Each district is divided with sub districts or taluks under which are situated community development blocks in the country. Adoption of the National Health Policy by both the Houses of Parliament has brought in a new turn. Health care programmes were restructured and reoriented towards this policy. Priority was given to extension and expansion of the rural health infrastructure through a net work of community health centres, primary health centres, and sub-centres on a liberalised population norm. Efforts were made to develop promotive and preventive services along with curative facilities. High priority was given to the development of primary health care located as close to the people as possible. Population norms have been revised to me one sub centre for 5000 population, community health centre for 30,000 and one community health centre health centre with four basic specialities for a population coverage of 1,00,000. District health organisation is to be strengthened to cater to the needs of the expanding rural health and family welfare programmes. Not only the planning and implementation and monitoring of health and family welfare programmes are to be cared out at the district level (preferably on a decentralised basis) but all the referral services from the periphery i.e. PHC community health centres and taluk hospitals are to be attended to satisfactorily.

III PHASE OF HEALTH TRANSITION

How can India enter the III phase and thereby achieve the goal of health for all by 2000 AD. III Phase is characterised by low mortality and low morbidity. In this connection one has to examine the factors which exercise profound influence on the health status.

It is natural to expect a rise in the health status of the people by increasing and improving the health facilities with more emphasis on the preventive aspect and rural health care as the new health policy levels stress on it.

Experience has shown that hospital based—disease-and-cure-oriented approach towards establishment of medical services has provided benefits only to those in the urban areas mostly and also has failed to achieve the goals in the field of health. Hence is the shift in emphasis to preventive promotive public health and rehabilitative aspects of the health care. Due attention must be paid to various aspects like nutritional status, prevention of food adulteration, maintenance of the quality of drugs, water supply, sanitation environmental protection, maternal and child health services, immunization, school health programmes, occupational health services, etc. The delivery systems also require to be properly evaluated periodically. The question of quality control and supervision have to be given importance in all schemes of evaluation. At the same time cost effective system of medicine like Ayurveda, unani, homeopathy etc. need to be encouraged. In this connection the importance of naturopathy is also worth mentioning. Every programme and policy which aims at enhancing the health status of the people must give due importance to rural areas. It may not be possible to set up one hospital in every village right now. Alternative must be thought off. For example, if we provide ambulance to each and every village to take the patient immediately to the hospital in the neighbourhood and if communication facilities are improved i.e. through telephone and than radio etc., it will be having great impact on the health status of the people.

ROLE OF EDUCATION

Mere provision of health facilities is not sufficient and there must be effective utilisation of these services and facilities offered. Here lies the role of education. Education and health both are complementary. They are the key components of human capital. If people are educated, there will be effective utilisation of the existing health care system and greater involvement of people in various health programmes which is aimed at in the new health policy. Health consciousness can be generated by educating people. Particularly in the rural areas people are afraid of immunization, they hesitate to use medical facilities and they depend on religious traits etc. Female literacy is a crucial factor which enables us to go nearer to the goal health for all by 2000 AD. Female literacy level definitely exercises profound influence on material mortality, infant mortality, child mortality, nutritional status and morbidity.

In this content it is worth mentioning about the recent article entitled 'Determinants of health status of people' by PH Reddy and Y.S. Gopal (Population centre, Bangalore). They have pointed out that the medical system comprising hospitals, doctors and drugs affects about 10 per cent of the health status of the people. The remaining 90 per cent is determined by factors over which medical system has little or no control. This means that a wide variety of factors like education food, nutrition, water, environmental sanitation and personal hygiene influence the health status of the people. Similar result has been obtained in our study also. We have collected time series data (A.P.) for fifteen years from 1970-85 for the following variables i.e. age specific death 2. number of hospitals and dispensaries, 3. number of doctors and 4. number of beds. We have selected an average figure for all ages—age specific death rate as the dependent variable and the remaining three variables as independent variables. We have found that the relationship between them is statistically significant but the impact of the explanatory variables is marginal.

Reddy and Gopal have considered health indicators and determinants of health status of the people for 21 states of India in 1981. Of the eight determinants female literacy turned out to be the most important determinant of health status. Female literacy ranked 1st in the case of both expectation of life at birth and crude death rate and ranked second with regard to infant mortality rate (Table 3).

We have tried to study the relationship between percentage of literacy and expectation of life in India during 1921-81 (Table 5). The correlation coefficient in the case of males is 0.97 and in the case of females it is 0.93. Hence it may be pointed out the spread of literacy must be paid due attention in the content of enhancement of health status.

Recent Human Development Report 1990 broughtout by the UNDP highlighted the importance of literacy while presenting the comparative profile of India, Pakistan and Sri Lanka (Table 5). The report pointed out that one of the most significant policy failures for India has been on the literacy front. From a 33 per cent adult literacy rate in 1970 after 15 years it has been risen only 43 per cent i.e. a municule growth rate of 0.97 per cent. Adult female literacy rates are even dismal. Female literacy has risen from 20 per cent in 1970 to only 29 per cent i.e. at a growth rate of 0.79 per cent. Pakistan illustrates what the report refers to as “missed opportunities for development”. Despite a higher income growth and relatively lower levels of poverty its diversion of scarce resources towards militarisation has been at the expense of education and health especially for women. On the other hand Sri Lanka reflects an alternative experience with higher levels of well-being despite a poor GNP, largely due to a long record of government intervention in the social sector. Literacy and particularly female literacy is much higher in Srilanka compared to India and Pakistan. Perhaps that may be the main reason for greater life expectancy is Srilanka.

CONCLUSION

Indeed an integrated approach is highly essential in order to achieve the goal of health for all by 2000 AD. Besides the expansion of health facilities (preventive and curative), one has to concentrate on various other factors like the spread of literacy, particularly female literacy; anti-poverty programmes, expanding employment opportunities; controlling inflation; effective implementation of family planning programme; provision of protected water supply in the rural areas and so on. A time bound programme with inter-sectoral cooperation and synchronisation of schemes and activities for the elimination of region specific local diseases etc. is needed. Synergic and dedicated efforts involving all the sectors, governmental agencies, voluntary organisations and the people would go a long way in effectively tackling promotive, preventive, curative, rehabilitative and emergency medicare and in translating the goal of "Health for all by 2000 AD" a living reality.

Table 1 : Health Services

	Item	*Unit*	*1950*	*1960*	*1971*	*1981*	*1984*
1.	Hospitals	1000	2.7	4.0	3.9	6.8	7.4
2.	Dispensaries	"	6.9	9.9	9.1	16.7	21.9
3.	Hospitals Beds	"	112	200	359	569	625
4.	Beds per lakh of population	No.	31	45	65	83	85
5.	Reg. Medical Practitioners	1000	59.3	76.0	148.5	268.7	295.8
6.	Reg. Medical Practitioners per lakh of population	No	17	18	27	39	40
7.	Regd. Names	1000	15.0	32.7	80.6	150.3	170.9

8.	Regd. Names per lakh of population	No.	4	8	15	22	23
9.	Medical Colleges	No.	29	87	98	106	106
10.	Annual admissions	100	2.5	10.6	12.1	10.7	11.1

Source : Ministry of Health and Family Welfare.

Table 2 : Vital Statistics 1951-81

INDIA

Vital rates	*1951*	*1961*	*1971*	*1981*	*1986*
Birth rate	39.9	41.7	49.0	35.9	32.4
Death rate	29.5	25.2	19.8	10.7	11.1
Infant Mortality rate	192	140	135	126	96
Child Mortality rate	76.27	59.06	55.48	48.26	—

Table 3 : Rankings of Selected Determinants Accordings to their importance for health indicators

Selected Determinants	*RANKINGS*		
	Expectation of life at Birth	*Infant Mortality Rate*	*Crude Death Rate*
Percentage of literates :			
Persons	2	3	3
Males	4	4	4
Females	1	2	1
Percentage of workers engaged in Non-agricultural activities	3	1	6
Female work participation rate	8	7	5
Percapita expenditure on health	6	5	2
Per capita net domestic product at current price	5	6	8
Percent of coupler effectively practising Family Planning	7	8	7

Source : "Determinants of Health Status of People" by P.H. Reddy & Y.S. Gopal Southern Economist, Aug. 15th 1997

Table 4 : Literacy and Expectation of Life 1901-1981

		% Literates to Total Population		*Expectation of life*	
Years	*Persons*	*Males*	*Females*	*Males*	*Females*
1901	5.3	9.8	0.7	23.6	24.0
1911	5.9	10.6	1.1	22.6	23.3
1921	7.2	12.2	1.8	19.4	20.9
1931	9.5	15.6	2.9	26.9	26.6
1941	16.1	24.9	7.3	32.1	31.04
1951	16.7	25.0	7.9	32.4	31.7
1961	24.0	34.4	13.0	41.9	40.6
1971	29.5	39.5	18.7	47.1	45.6
1981	36.2	46.9	24.8	52.62	51.55

Table 5 : Comparative Profile : India, Pakistan and Srilanka

		India	*Pakistan*	*Srilanka*
1.	Adult Literacy (1985 in %age)	43	30	87
2.	Adult literacy male	57	40	91
3.	Adult literacy Female	29	19	83
4.	Life Expectancy at birth (1987)	59	58	71
5.	Maternal mortality (1980-87) for one lakh life births	340	500	60
6.	Population with access to safe drinking water (%) (1985-87)	57	44	40
7.	Ratio of military expenditure to health and education expenditure (1986)	81	279	116
8.	Armed Forces as % of teachers (1986)	28	154	12
9.	G N P rankin	25	33	38
10.	H D I ranking	26	37	3

13

EDUCATION, AGE AT MARRIAGE AND FAMILY PLANNING

Dr. Viswanatham Kanithi

1. India's National Health Policy envisages "HEALTH FOR ALL BY 2000 A.D." It is possible only when the Government, Dept. of Health, Voluntary Organisations and Public, work together to achieve the set goal.

   A. All systems of medicine in practice in India must be given the due share to participate.

   B. All nook and corners of the country must be covered by a chain of Health Service Centres. Basic bare foot Health Workers, Primary Health Centres, Base level Taluk Hospitals, District Head Quarters Hospitals and Referral Medical Institutions must work in coordination for Health Education, immunisation and Small Family norm.

2. Population growth is enormous in India leading to explosion. All concerned parties, Government, Political parties, Health Dept., Education Department, Voluntary organisations must take it up seriously or else the expected peace and harmony that is expected during the coming years of development will be a Myth. At the time of independence in 1947 our population was put at 33 crores and now it is galloping leaps and bounds to cross 83 crores in 90s and 100 crores in 2000 A.D. The yearly growth is equal to the whole population of Australia which is much bigger than India. The rate of growth is put at 24/1000 staggeringly reduced from 36/thousand 1950.

The aim of growth is less than 10/thousand. The target must be negative growth—6/thousand.

The Government of India has officially declared to adopt Small family norm in 1950 and various steps were taken in these 40 long years and the results are not encouraging for various reasons—illiteracy, religion, superstition, lack of awareness of the gravity of the situation by both the rulers and ruled; lack of dedicated personnal at the grass-root level to motivate and the disparity in offering incentives to the acceptors from Artisan to Officer. All these put together, has led to marriages before attaining the age of 20 years. By 21 we expect a person, especially a female gets the ability to decide what to do, how to do and how many number of children to bear, if married, depending upon the earning capacity.

As on date the present programme has come to a stand still. You may be surprised to note that the present plan of action is ineffective according to people, in high office. A change is most welcome and needed. It shall certainly be effective if it is innovative and useful.

While keeping all the drawbacks and kickbacks, in view, and rectifying the defects and deficiencies, let us tackle the main problem—illiteracy among female folk of the have nots. As we all known that the upper class of the present day society could educate their children male and female, till the age of 20 years and upwards and so much so they are following the small family norm to a great extent. So you may take the clue that education of all females of 5-20 age groups upto the age of 20 by all possible means. We all know this is a gigantic project. There is nothing like an easy way for success—except hard and sincere work.

I would like to suggest that all the eligible girls must be picked up and made then to enrole in the respective class in Elementary Schools. If necessary average mid day meal or subsidy to the parents—which will replace the usual nominal income earned by the girls in the low income group. Keep them in schools for 12 hours making them active not only in education but also in other extra curricular activities of their choice, which can make the student feel encouraged and interested. In the latter years of schooling the students can be subjected to special courses like vocational training which can give a sense of self-reliance and confidence in real life, that she too can play her part for the Nation building through Technical Education, Professional education and vocational training in 150 varieties, available with labour training and employment Government of India in the country.

If this can be implemented starting with those below poverty line, we can go a long way.

Just like the way we have special residential schools for S.C. & S.Ts. We can as well run such Residential Schools for girls of those who need, especially form the families below the poverty line, if not all the eligible girls. If every thing said is done we can reach the goals in 15 years from the date of take off.

Religion plays a part in attaining Small Family Norm. All the Religious heads of the Country the States and Regions must be taken into confidence, inspired, motivated to follow and adopt the laws of the land equally. No religion or sect is above board for advocation or otherwise of the programme of the Nation. Positive and negative incentives can lure the Target couples.

Superstition was one of the reasons for failure of the programme and now it is slowly vanishing. Education and motivation alone can solve the problem. All people especially the teen aged students, youth and target couple must be made aware of the need of the small family norm, through curriculum, seminars, daily press reports, Radio, T.V. advertisements and wall paintings throughout the country.

Voluntary individuals in Service and outside service and organisations must be welcomed to form local and regional forums and assist and coordinate their work with the authorities. Service organisations when involved can create a sense of confidence in the people as seen in Cataract operations camps conducted by Service organisations.

If the Government can go to the extent of asking the person incharge of Family Planning to join the Service Organisation and inspire and encourage, the Family Planning work can catch up quicker momentum.

Monetary incentives must be equal to all acceptors at all times. No exception—either to the poor, rich, employed or unemployed in the country. If the Government wants to give extra incentives it must be given first to those below the poverty line. The multiplication among people below poverty line, is making the country poorer and poorer. For any programme of long duration frequent changes and innovative methods, can give a new direction, impetus and fillup to the programme.

As an example : for immediate results not waiting for 15 or more years, it is the lower strata of people who are adding new mouths every year, they can be offered a luring and attractive financial assistance like a Rs. 50,000/- bond non transferable, non encashable before the fixed date of 21 years for on the date of death; Rs. 3,000/- Bond issued at the time of Family Planning operation and where the child is one year old, this amount will become Rs. 50,000/- at maturity of the bond a suitable amount to reckon with. It can be used for the self employment of the grown up youth—give them an identity Nomination card and the Bond.

Family Planning Methods : No particular method used in Family Planning is fool proof. We have temporary and permanent methods.

As of the temporary methods :

1. Pill is not universally accepted and spotless.
2. Gellies and Foams could not make a dent.
3. Condom (F.L.) unacceptable by illiterate and it encourages adultery.
4. Pessay, loop and copper-T have not been successful in all cases.
5. Flexible ring is giving good results.
6. Hormones implants and Tablets are costly and not free of trouble making.
7. Vasectomy in males is the best and trouble free method.
8. Tubectomy properly done—Button hole Tubectomy in its true sense, is innovative and simple, the best method if properly done under specific conditions and is the safest one.
9. His Tubectomy after two children produces 2 birds for 1 shot. (no children no cancer to uterus cervix).
10. If ovaries are exposed to deep X rays for short time, can produce not only sterility but also other complications like imbalance in hormones.
11. Oral consumption of an Ayurvedic medicine is giving good results. Trails and experimentations are going on. Let us wait and see for the final result.

For Immediate results:

The operative procedures can be conducted meticulously on a war footing. For chosen area, we must have three teems selected from voluntary individuals chosen for the purpose for a particular term or long term service.

1st Team consists of youth from Colleges, N.S.S., N.C.C., service organisations and Government and Health Dept., who goes to the villages and towns, makes a survey, fixes up targets and motivate them and acceptor lists are prepared and handed over to 2nd Team— which operates 10 to 30 cases a day by a single team with special training, and proceeds to another (3rd team) leaving a Doctor or responsible person incharge of the operated cases till such time his presence is no longer needed and the sutures are removed. It any complication arises the case can be brought to the nearest Health Care Centre or Hospital. This act shall instill the confidence in the acceptor, which is lacking hitherto. It is is taken up seriously on a country wide basis with all the infrastructure keeping on hand, we can cover the entire country in 3 years. Afterwards the new T.C. will follow predecessors.

To conclude (1) the college students and the educated unemployed can be associated with the Government and the Service Organisations for survey and motivation. They can also be utilised for illiteracy eradication programme and awareness. (2) The unemployed Doctors can be employed on short term basis to associate with specially trained surgeons who can operate and entrust the follow up. (3) Innovative and luring incentives like long term maturable cash certificates with insurance cover can certainly give a big bang (4) Equal and uniform cash incentives throughout the country to all acceptors (5) Residential Schooling to all School age group children or atleast to all girls of the weaker sections and those below poverty line with an emphasis on imparting need based self employment oriented education upto the age of 20 years can certainly raise the marriageable age of the woman of poorer sections who are the factors for populations rapid growth since the educated upper classes women are marrying around 20. It may be noted that with the introduction of Residential Schools for Girijans the percentage of educated among that age group has increased considerably during last five years (6) Simultaneously implementation of both long term and short term methods to check the population growth is a must. (7) All Government and Non-Government Departments and concerns must encourage the scheme, adopt the villages and areas of the urban localities to implement plan projects with devotion and dedication ..... EACH ONE REACH ONE.

SECTION D

MANAGEMENT OF HEALTH SECTOR

14

HEALTH MANAGEMENT — A SYSTEMS APPROACH

Professor M. Chandrasekhar and Sri. P. Balaji Prasad

Health is wealth. Health is a total concept, which includes preventive, promotive, curative and rehabilitative. According to WHO, "Health is a state of complete physical, mental and social well-being not merely the absence of disease or infirmity". Thus, health of individuals is the wealth of nations.

In view of the above, taking care of the health of individual is not only the concern of individuals but also the concern of health institutions sponsored by Government, voluntary and private organisations. The management of health care at individual, organisational, national and international level is of great concern. Recognising human beings as an important resource the human resource management has become a significant a field of activity.

There are several forces responsible for growing concern on health care management. The health care planning started in 1937. After Independence health care in India was directed by constitution. Accordingly, "State shall regard the raising of the level of nutrition and the standard of living of the people and the improvement of public health as among it's primary duties. Behind this back drop, the health, hospitals, medical services are developed through the five year plans. The plan investment on health has increased from Rs. 65.20 crores, in 1951-56 to Rs. 1821 crores during 1980-85. However, the percentage of investment in health to total plan outlay dropped from 3.3 per cent in the first plan to 1.86 per cent in Sixty Plan as indicated in Table 1.

Table 1 : Investment in Health in Relation to Total Plan outlay in five year plans

S. No.	*Plan Period*	*Total plant outlay (Rs. in crores)*	*Plant investment on health (Rs. in crores)*	*Investment in health in relation to total plan outlay*
1	2	*3*	*4*	*5*
First Plan	1951-56	1,960.00	65.20	3.3
Second Plan	1956-61	4,672.00	140.80	3.0
Third Plan	1961-66	8,576.50	225.90	2.6
Annual Plan	1966-69	6,625.40	140.20	2.1
Fourth Plan	1969-74	15,778.80	140.20	2.1
Fifth Plan	1974-78	39,426.20	760.80	1.9
Annual Plan	1978-80	12,176.50	223.10	1.82
Sixth Plan	1980-85	97,500.00	1821.10	1.86

Source : INDIA 1985 : Ministry of Information and Broadcasting, Government of India, New Delhi.

From the above, though there is an increase in planned allocation to health in absolute terms, there is a decline, in relation to total plan outlay. This indicates the scaling down of priority to health sector in preference to others.

The annual per capita distribution of investment as indicated in Table 2 was 34 paise in 1951-56 when the population was around 380 millions. However, it increased during the successive five year plans and it was around five rupees with the population of 727 millions in 1980-85. Though the increase on per capita distribution is appreciated, the allocations made were nullified in real terms with the escalating cost over runs in the economy over the period. Further, with the increased life expectancy over the period the demand for health care has increased manifold. The renewed emphasis on human resources would not carry any conviction without giving adequate priority for health support systems in budget. It within the existing system there is going to be budgetary constraints, there is need to generate additional resources to facilitate health promotion systems.

Table 2 : Per Capita Investment in Health

S. No.	*Plan Period*	*Plant investment on health (Rs. in crores)*	**Population during the period (in million)*	*Per capita distribution on health (in Rs./annum)*
1	*2*	*3*	*4*	*5*
First Plan	1951-56	65.20	380	0.34
Second Plan	1956-61	140.80	420	0.66
Third Plan	1961-66	225.90	465	0.97
Annual Plan	1966-69	140.20	504	0.92
Fourth Plan	1969-74	335.40	555	1.20
Fifth Plan	1974-78	760.80	623	2.43
Annual Plan	1978-80	223.10	657	1.69
Sixth Plan	1980-85	1821.10	727	5.00

Source : Compiled and calculated based on information in INDIA 85, Ministry of Information and Broadcasting, Government of India.

* : The Population for respective plan period was kept constant for calculation purpose. Where population coincide with census, it was taken as it is. But for other plan periods it is arrived by calculating growth rate for the respective decades.

Another pointer of concern is pattern of expenditure of the medical budget. It was estimated that about 80 per cent of the medical budget is being spent on 20 per cent of the people living in urban areas. This coupled with drop of allocation of funds to health in relation to total outlay from 3.3 per cent to 1.86 per cent has increased health problems of the vast multitudes people living in making rural people to look to urban areas for better medical facilities and is forcing them to incur more incidental changers like expenses for travelling, accommodation, food and other expenses than the actual health costs.

In terms of coverage of the health facilities, we had the shortfalls as can be observed from some of the following facts. As against the WHO recommendation of one health centre for every 20000 population we could achieve one health centre for 40000 population. Bed facilities in the hospitals recommended was two beds for every one thousand population. But so far we had achieved 0.7 bed for one thousand population by the end of Sixth Plan. Doctor per 5100 population. However, there are places with one doctor for nearly 50000 population. If we have to meet those standards there is need to study the alternative ways of improving the set health targets.

Within the existing health care infrastructure developed so far there are several imbalances. Hospitals are generally under employed to the growing demands. The skills, attitudes, the knowledge of the medical and paramedical staff are significant in health seminars. The best trained and motivated people are in short supply to the cause of public health service. With medical talent being unavailable to the public service, and the available medical talent in the service being unable to meet growing demand, there is a growing medical unemployment on one hand and growing demand for basic as well as the quality medical care on the other. Very often hospitals are ill equipped in terms of medicines and other equipments. With the above scenario, people are getting a raw deal in the hospitals. Thus, there is a need for re-examination of health policies at all levels. The ever increasing population, environmental pollution, rapid industrialisation and irregular urbanisation also have greater impact on health and health maintenance. Hence, changes contemplated must also take note of above developments.

So far the role of people in the health care system is that of passive recipients. The system is impervious to people's influence. Any public task without people's active participation is going to be a difficult one to succeed. Hence the health care system must involve people in preventive care, dissemination of medical and health education, and making system a viable one. But the people's role must be in the nature of participative and problem solving. Further, this should facilitate promotion and monitoring of health system to the growing and changing needs. Thus there is a need for best people's participation in health maintenance and distribution systems.

In view of the above, there is every need to strengthen health sector both financially and managerially by redesigning the organisation structure with improved technological and information inputs and participation of all concerned.

URBAN HEALTH

There is a general inadequacy of Primary Health Care. It must be noted that primary health care and rural health care are not synonymous. A cost effective institutional based approach may be more appropriate in urban areas while an extension-based approach relevant for rural health services.

USER CHARGES

Currently, the government hospitals provide nearly free services to all. Government is also concerned about coverage and affordability of the poor. There is a need to institute user charges on a differential basis, i.e. free for people below the poverty line (a level which is recognised by the state) subsidised for some other income brackets, and finally higher than full costs to higher income brackets. Appropriate studies should lead to fixing up the cost structure, ensuring reference generation.

The Health-card system is yet another alternative which can be explored. It is recognised at policy making levels that a fee-for-service system can lead to improved utilisation patterns and current to a certain extent the malfunctioning of intended referral system.

PRIVATE CURATIVE CARE

With the increases standard of living, responsive policy and rapid advancements in medical technology. The private health care sector is fast expanding. This call for coordination between the public and private sector. Firstly government should avoid duplication and use services as referral for poor patients in return for concessions. Secondly the concessions so granted should be geographically dispersed and equitable. A policy on the role of private territory care and its regulatory framework needs to be developed.

For the secondary care facility network, a health care financing mechanism/fund agency should be promoted for encouraging development of cooperative hospitals and evolving appropriate insurance packages.

Regarding the rural health care, in order to influence health status, there is need for more emphasis on staff, material equipment, training and development rather then on buildings. The referral system has to be made effective.

HEALTH INSURANCE

There is tremendous potential for this in the country. There are examples like a rural based scheme in Maharashtra, insurance linked medical benefit scheme in Calcutta called SEBA. Encouraging insurance policies of State owned companies such as General Insurance Company. As a good social security measure, schemes like Employee State Insurance scheme, though there are some operational difficulties in its implementation. The amount of cash benefits given to the insured persons is very substantial.

HOUSEHOLD EXPENDITURE ON HEALTH CARE

One of the important components of expenditure on medical and health services is the expenditure incurred by the households in making direct payments for doctors, medicines and other medical services. The per capita per/month household expenditure data from the 1977-78 based on NSSO surveys is an estimated expenditure elasticity of health and medical care was significant. A one per cent increases in the per capita total expenditure would lead to an increase of more than the proportion of their income on health and medical care services. Therefore, there is greater need to channelise the source of income for the augmentation of health care services.

COST REDUCTION

There is a greater need to innovate and intime in the aspect of health care services, government hospitals, expenditure on communicable disease control, rational plans for health facilities in the government as well as private sector. They should be developed after a careful epidemiological and locational analysis.

HEALTH INFORMATION SYSTEM (HIS)

Due to inadequate collection, maintenance and analysis of disaggregated cost data administrators are unable to comprehend alternatives even though many have indicated their felt-need for such as information system for financial planning and management.

Thus one of the important issues is to first develop a system of data collection, maintenance, analysis for taking decisions pricing, resource allocations between programmes, effective cost control measures and improving efficiency of programme implementation.

Before attempting to rationalise the health care systems, there is need to concentrate on the pre-requisite of developing an appropriate data base.

BIBLIOGRAPHY

1. John Laplace, 'Health', Appleton Century Crofts, New York.
2. India 1985 Year Book, Reference Manual—Ministry of I & B, Government of India.
3. Dr. DRF Pinto 'Hospital Planning', Indian Management, November '87.
4. SN Chaudhuri, 'Health based development' Decision, October, 1979.
5. Dr. Ashok Sahni—"Seventh Plan projections—Health Management Issues", Indian Management, November 1987, p. 8-11.

15

SELECTIVE PRIMARY HEALTH CARE (A CASE OF UNIVERSAL IMMUNISATION PROGRAMME)

Dr. K.N. Kondala Rao

Essential health care based on practical, scientifically sound and socially acceptable methods and technology made universally accessible to individuals and families in the community through their full participation and at a cost that the community and the country can afford to maintain at every stage of their development in the spirit of self-determination.

HEALTH FOR ALL BY 2000 AD

This goal is the attainment by all the people of the world by the year 2000 AD of a level of health that will permit them to lead a Socially and Economically productive life. It means that there will be an even distribution among the population of whatever resources for health are availables so that people will use the available approaches for better health. It implies wide ranging improvements not only in access to health services, but parallel, social and economic development.

Alma Ata declaration (WHO'78) is an important watershed in the history of public health. It advocates formation of systems of health services that are built around the people rather than around technology—to guage people response and to promote community self-reliance. Health services are under social control as an component of wider intersectoral action for health improvement.

But the affluent countries came forward with selective primary health care, a technocentric dependence producing approach. It is a contradiction to the concept of Primary Health Care. It lacks scientific basis. But it received support from UNICEF launching the child survival development revolution.

Many scholars expressed deep concerned over this obvious attempts. Public health experts at Antwerp Institute of Tropical Medicine declared in 1985 as

> "..... in developing countries inspite of the lessons of history and of past experience, major national and international donar agencies are divertising scare resources into a short-term approach known as selective primary health care. This approach concentrates exclusively on certain interventions claimed to be the most efficient and aimed only at sections of the population. This self-contradictory term should be banned since at their best, such programmes can only be considered as selective health status interventions. This approach is in total contradiction with the fundamental principles underlying Primary Health Care.

The earlier EPI is converted into U.I.P., made more selective. Debabar Banerji, stated that while the protection of children in consonance with broad-based primary health care activities is a desirable objective the immunisation package being promoted today ignores vital epidemilogical, biological and administrative factors.

Health improvements brought about by GOBI, can only be sustained by the availability of food, water and shelter and the political and economic power of the people to obtain them. Questions are opened on the motivation behind the efforts to impose technocentric approaches to deal with the problems of child health in the third world, though the problems are routed in the ecological conditions prevailing in these countries. The flaws are :

1. Massive expensive and complicated programmes.
2. Epidemilogical consideration are ignored such as incidents rates, ecological conditions and the time-trends of the chosen diseases.
3. Other Critical areas : Efficacy of different strains of vaccines, storage, mode of vaccine administration, maintenance of cold chain, fixation of the level of herd immunity, impact of the time-bound, target oriented programme on health services etc.

India has set up Indo-U.S. vaccine action project (GOI), 1982. U.I.P. envisaged an expenditure of 250 crores (G.O.I. '85). It was a gigantic takes. From April, 1985, within 5 years more than 90 million pregnant mothers and 83 million infants living in more than 5,75,000 villages were to be immunised. It required 30,00,000 vaccine careers, 15.2 million syringes, 60 million needles and over 1,000 million doses of vaccines. In addition, the stupendous problems are concerning vaccine production, import of vaccines and equipment, ensuring timely supplies, cold chain, promoting community participation, education and communication, training and monitoring evaluation and surveillance. It is an impossible task in states as Uttar Pradesh, Bihar, Rajasthan, Madhya Pradesh, Orissa, Assam and West-Bengal to administer this due to work organisational structures at the periphery an even the weaker management system. Also U.I.P. damages other activities like the National T.B. Programme. In states accounting for more than the half of the population of country, less than a fifth of the eligible children were fully protected against the five diseases. Even in the best performance states the coverage is not the prescribed 85%. The states are Kerala, Himachal Pradesh and Goa (U.T.). These states already had low mortality and morbidity rates and the impact of the coverage will be limited.

Hence the question is not of rejection of all technology but to ensure that concerned efforts are made to promote self-reliance and to sub-ordinate technology to the needs of the people as contained in the Alma Ata Declaration.

REFERENCES

1. Text book of Social and preventive medicine, J.E. Park.
2. Seminar magazines.
3. New England Journal of Medicine, Vol. 30.

16

NEED FOR NEW POLICIES AND PROGRAMMES FOR HEALTH PROMOTION IN INDIA

K. Mahadevan, M. Ubaidullah and Azuh Dominic Ezinwa

INTRODUCTION

India is one of the backward countries in the field of promotion of health and control of population among several nations in Asian continent. India (IMR 106) along with Bangladesh (IMR 135) and Pakistan (IMR 124) have the highest level of infant mortality and crude birth rate of over 14 and 35 respectively compared to the rest of Asian Countries by 1983. India also has one of the highest (CDR 14) incidence of general mortality compared to the most successful countries in Asia viz., Singapore (CDR 5), Hong Kong (CDR 5), Thailand (CDR 7), Srilanka (CDR 6), Taiwan (CDR 5), South Korea (CDR 8), Malaysia (CDR 7) and China (CDR 8) in the Asian continent. Also India's birth rate (CBR) remains at much higher level (32 now) as against that of Singapore (CBR 17), Hong Kong (CBR 17), Taiwan (CBR 23), Srilanka (CBR 28), China (CBR 23), Thailand (CBR 28), Malaysia (CBR 31) and South Korea (CBR 32). The life expectancy at birth in India (59) was one of the third lowest along with Bangladesh (47) and Pakistan (58) compared to other progressive Asian countries mentioned above (Population References Bureau, 1983).

In the light of the preceding information given, it is encouraging and rewarding for India to gain experiences from most of these Asian countries for making rapid strides in the field of health and population control programmes, instead of following the stero-typed policies and programmes which continue to make this country backward in these areas.

However, a comparison of India's programme with Malaysia alone revealed the lopsided development of Indian health and family planning programmes leading to the present plight of poor health status of the people and rapid growth of population in India. For want of time and space the comparison is not extended to other Asian countries.

HIGHER INVESTMENT IN HEALTH AND POPULATION IS NEEDED

During the Seventh Five Year Plan periods, a range of 5-7 per cent of the total investment under different plan periods was made for the promotion of various health and family planning programmes in India. Under the Seventh Plan period alone 7.3 per cent of the plan allocation was spent for the health and family welfare programmes. It includes 1.9 per cent for health, 1.8 per cent for family welfare and 3.6 per cent for water supply and sanitation respectively. No doubt, this amount needs to be raised considerably in view of the existing over 800 million population, poor infrastructural facilities, poverty, miserable sanitation and poor health and social-backwardness of the population in general. While a small country like Malaysia could spend 25 per cent of their budget for the promotion of this programme, we hardly spent only one third of that amount in the field of most backward areas of social development. Compared to most of the other Asian countries.

A comparison of the GNP between India and Malaysia shows that our GNP is only US $ 253 as against US $ 1,817 for Malaysia (PRB, 1983; Rahimah, 1990). In other words, the GNP of India is less than 1/7 of Malaysia. Under normal circumstances, India should have spent more money for health and family planning as compared to Malaysia. As a result of the differential investment made for health and family planning by two developing countries of Asia viz., India and Malaysia, the former is facing one of the highest incidence of infant mortality (IMR 122, General Mortality (CDR 15) high fertility (CBR 32) and a lower level of longevity (59) in contrast to very low infant mortality (IMR 31), general mortality (CDR 7), low birth rate (CBR 31), and relatively high level of longevity (life expectancy at birth 64) for Malaysia.

Since the characteristics of population of Malaysia and India are quite similar in the field of ethnicity, religion, duration of independence and level of development at the time of attaining freedom, the present significant differences noticed in the field of health and population growth, could be largely due to differential investment made for these programmes in these countries. The preceding comparison of financial input and health and population output underlines the urgent necessity for giving higher allocation of finance during the 8th plan period for the promotion of health and family planning in India.

MAXIMISE THE UTILISATION OF EXISTING FACILITIES

The past experiences of utilisation of the existing infrastructural facilities in rural areas in India may have been very shocking for planners and administrators. For the country as a whole, not even 25 per cent of the existing infrastructural facilities in both rural and urban areas have been utilised by the people for promoting health and limiting family size. When the country spend over Rupees Twelve thousand crores approximately for health and population alone during a recent Five Year Plan period for the benefit of the entire population and this much investment was made use of by only a 1/4 of the total population, we can imagine the colossal waste which exists for the investment already made in this programme. Therefore, equal priority may be given for increasing future investment along with the necessary steps to ensure that the major part of population uses the existing facilities. Otherwise the benefit of the investment of resources will be wasted. What can be done for maximising the use of the existing facilities is a major concern and the focus of attention of this paper.

Utilisation of the existing facilities for health and population is one of the highest in Kerala State, where it is as high as 80 per cent in contrast to less than 25 per cent in Andhra Pradesh and less than 10 per cent in the Gangetic plains. The greater utilisation of short distances in most of the rural areas, extensive network of road and transport facilities, favourable worker-population ratio, enlightenment of the population and empowerment of clients through education and modernization and so on (Mahadevan and Sumangala, 1987). Kerala invested more than Malaysia for the health and population programmes, and also for education. Their total investment in these two major fields of social development was very much closer to 40 per cent of the total investment of the government. Why cannot the rest of the states in India take the clue from the successful experiences of Kerala, Malaysia, Thailand, Srilanka, Taiwan, South Korea and China for the rapid reduction in mortality and fertility? Therefore, the 8th Plan should give a greater thrust for maximising the utilization of the existing facilities. In this context a few policy issues have been considered in this paper.

Guidance counter : For maximising the use of the existing facilities in most of the hospitals, a health educator/nurse or a compounder, who have been trained effectively in human relations should receive a patient with a smile, screen him/her for different types of treatment and refer the client suitably to the units concerned. This procedure will go a long way in minimising frustration and difficulties of the patient and bridging the gap of acceptability between the clients and the doctors effectively. Such a procedure does not exist even in many popular and reputed medical colleges and hospitals. To give an example, it is frustrating to get registration for a medical check-up, even in a reputed medical college like Vellore, where the patient has to go from one booth to another for 2-3 hours to complete the cumbersome procedure. It can be simplified for the satisfaction of the client if a proper reception cell is established in most of the major hospitals and medical colleges. Similar innovations may have to be considered for improving the service facilities in order to maximise their utility.

Expansion of Out-reach : During the last 42 years, the independent India promoted health and population control through the government-owned Primary Health Centres and sub-centres. Though the principle is laudable for rendering these services freely, the benefit has not reached the overwhelming proportion of population in rural areas. Consequently, nearly 80 per cent of the investment male so far in this sector remained unutilised. Should we continue to be prisoners of this ideological obsession? Is it not the time to have a re-thinking to change the delivery of peripheral health services? Why not involve the non-government agencies to serve in remote areas by providing them with loans and incentives to set up clinics in order to bridge the gap of service facilities? In addition, should we not ask the existing medical colleges in this country numbering over 150 to extend their services to one district each in and around their location? Is it justifiable for these medical colleges to remain as ivory towers limiting their minimum services to in-patients and negligible number of out-patients alone? Millions of rupees have been spent for establishing each medical college and is it not their duty to serve effectively at least in one district each?

The present institutionalised delivery of health services expecting the clients to visit hospitals and receive treatment should be reversed and insteads at least two out of three or four doctors in a Primary Health Centre be made to visit remote villages to extend services at the doorstep of the people. Unless a reversal of the services and programmes from institution-oriented service to community-oriented service is adopted, the existing negligible utilisation of hospitals will continue to remain for decades. This new pattern of health delivery system may be supported during the 8th plan period for its effectively utilisation.

Improve worker-population ratio : Health-worker population ratio in India is one of the most disadvantageous aspects of the administrative set up compared to the situation prevailing in most of the other Asian countries, not to speak of the developed countries. When India's population doubled during the last 42 years after independence, health worker-population ratio in India hardly doubled during the same period. Even if they were tripled during the last 4 decades it would not have been sufficient considering the *poor infrastructural facilities, inadequate transport, low level of literacy and negligible demand for the existing modern health facilities.* Although during the 7th Plan period a policy dection was made to trifurcate the existing development blocks into 3 PHC zones, this policy has not been translated into action in most of the Indian states. While Kerala state in India has a Allopathic and Ayurvedic hospitals each in every major village which has revolutionalised the health facilities to most of the population in rural areas, most of the other villages in India do not have such facilities.

For bridging the gap of service on health delivery system, in addition to the existing full-time government staff *more part-time staff can be appointed on a large scale* to give employment to educated people and also to meet the growing needs of the vast majority of the population with available resources. It is not advisable to appoint, after short term training, unemployed educated youths particularly girls on a part time basis with moderate salary for the next five years and in a phased manner and absorbed them into regular service till the government generates sufficient resources? Such efforts will be more rewarding than giving unemployment allowance to *youths* as has been done in Kerala and Tamil Nadu. When partially trained youths are employed for health and family planning programme they can be fully trained in the long run through the existing 46 Regional Health and Family Welfare Training Centres (which are under utilised now), 150 medical colleges and other nursing schools. Such efforts may minimise unemployment and meet the growing needs of health and family planning service facilities. In fact they should be used as agents of change in promoting health education and population control programme. Given sufficient incentives and encouragement besides giving periodic in-service training they can help to deliver the goods on proper lines.

Inter-sectoral Co-ordination : Although considerable improvement has been made in India for establishing hospitals at the peripheral level, taluk level and at the district besides the medical colleges and also transport facilities, telephone and other communication facilities, negligible co-ordination exists between transport agencies, department of communication and hospital service timings. While in developed countries they have air line facilities to transport patients in helicopters from remote areas to specialised hospitals during a very short span of time, we do not have even elementary facilities to transport patients from remote areas to nearby PHCs, even by ordinary vehicle, not to speak of metropolitan hospitals and referral hospitals. This is the major snag in the inter-sectoral co-ordination in maximising the existing service facilities. *If we have telephone facilities in every village, connecting transport facilities from villages to hospitals during working hours, most of the hospitals could have been used effectively.* In addition, to this inter-sectoral co-operation, the existing mass media also should co-operate in announcing the availability of expert facilities in different places and in popularising modern hospital services and at the same time educating the public about the dangers of using the services of indigenous quacks. Thus, a number of agencies viz., hospitals (Government and Private), transport agencies, telecommunication, mass media like newspaper, radio and television etc., may have to work in a co-ordinated manner to improve the utilisation of the existing health service facilities. Unfortunately, today these agencies do not have any form of co-ordinated service for the common good of the people. They all work independently on their own lines. There are many more such agencies who may have to be involved for maximising the use of the existing facilities and for this purpose new studies are needed to identify the nature and extent of inter-sectoral co-operation for promotion of health in remote areas.

Compulsory health and sex education for all : Although the basic purpose of education is to improve the quality of life of the population, the present education in India does not meet this requirement sufficiently. The present day's subject and curriculum taught in different classes in the undergraduate programme have paid seant regard for improving the quality of the population. For improving subjects like environmental sanitation, checking different types of pollution and their hazards to health, promoting importance of personal hygiene, nutrition education health and population education and protection of the eco-system in general are the high priority subjects. It is surprising that these subjects are not taught for children in schools and colleges. Instead subjects of lower priority including Civics and Social Studies are imparted to students at the neglect of these essential subjects. Such subjects can be learned informally through newspapers, but subjects on quality of life cannot be easily understood through mass media because of their technical nature and inadequate media coverage of these subjects at present.

It is a matter of shamc that people who have secured doctoral degrees in India on several social science subjects are ignorant of human physiology, methods of prevention of diseases and even the elementary first-aid needed for averting risks from epidemics and many communicable diseases. What purpose will be served with such education without simultaneous knowledge of health education for a better quality of life? Therefore, there is urgent necessity to introduce a compulsory paper on health education with the essential subjects mentioned above right from the elementary school level to the Higher Secondary level. In addition, this subject should form a major focus of adult education and non-formal education to non-school going children and adults because of the heavy drop-out of children from schools.

Sex education should be at a high priority level in health education in India in the context of growing adolescent pregnancies, increasing abortion rate, spread of Veneral Diseases and the dreadful AIDS. Although teenage pregnancy is very rare in India compared to USA and Denmark, where one out of every 10 teenage girls of the age group of 14-19 becomes pregnant. Statistics in India for this is inadequate but the per cent will not be even what we see in USA and Denmark. Although parents and close relatives transmit message on sex to teenaged girls and boys, it is a sensitive issue for them to do it. "Public opinion polls in USA has strongly shown support for sex education including birth control information to children from class 6th onwards". The content of sex education increases from the 9th class onwards. If sex education is introduced on a limited scale to school going and out of school teenagers, it may greatly supplement and simplify the efforts needed for family planning in future. In addition, it may improve the health status of women, reduce maternal morbidity and mortality of women (Rosoff, 1989).

"In all the developing countries, teenagers experience greater maternal mortality and morbidity than women over the age of 20 for a combination of biological and social reasons. In addition, children born to adolescent mothers are less likely to survive than those born to mothers are less likely to survive than those born to mothers who are over age 20. Women who begin child-bearing at early ages are more likely to be poorer and less educated than those who postpone child-bearing to later ages. Responses to the problem of adolescent fertility in developed countries focus on sex eduction and contraception for adolescents. Therefore, a UN report concluded "Sex education for young people is provided through schools' curricula in some countries, but the content often does not include education about pregnancy prevention because of opposition by those who believe that such knowledge fosters sexual activity. Moreover, in most developing countries, the majority of girls do not reach secondary schools where sex education in usually given" (UN, 1989).

The curriculum for health education in schools and colleges should be modified to include the precautions to be given for the young people in their life-style like use of condom to prevent AIDS, suitable exercise including yoga for the health of every organ in the body, appropriate dietary pattern and for prevention of gerontological diseases later on. In addition, even the seating arrangements of boys and girls in schools and colleges must be planned to prevent them from being physically handicapped and affecting the proper growth of the body system. The curriculum should also contain essential contents for unlearning the wrong habits and customs and reinforcing it with new scientific life-style for the health of every organ in the body.

NEW PERSPECTIVES ON HUMAN RESOURCE DEVELOPMENT

The service at the PHCs and hospitals by the doctors and paramedicals requires comprehensive education for them in their respective courses. When the doctor spends fifty per cent of his/her time for administering the activities of the hospital, he/she hardly learns anything in management skill from his graduate programme. In addition, should the technically qualified personnel like a doctor waste his time in administration instead of fully devoting it is curative and preventive services? Is it not time to restructure the curriculum and staff partner on a realistic basis? In their training programme itself there is need to educate them to prevent wastage which is a general feature now in hospitals and improve the human relations between the provider and the clients.

Today while most of the PHC doctors remain partially or fully idle during the limited period of a couple of hours at the PHC in the mornings, most of the quacks and indigenous physicians are very busy and over working. Why does such a paradoxical situation exist between the trained doctors and quack in rural areas ? The Simple answer for this is that the quack as an individual manifests pleasant human relation with the clients which is absent in the government doctors. When the same PHC doctor conducts a private clinic, he manifests excellent human relation with the clients. Therefore, is it hypocrisy in service or is there something else wrong in the process, or is it a defect of the administration itself? Therefore, a thorough review of the human resource development of different categories of workers and administrative procedure are urgently needed to save the health delivery system from its gross under utilisation.

Another very important aspect for maximising the utilisation of the existing facility is to improve the quality and image of the service centre. In this context, the procedure in the hospital should not be cumbersome as stated earlier and time consuming. For instance, a patient has to spend six to eight hours in a general hospital to pass through the various counters of different departments and points of check-up before he or she gets a prescription for treatment. For the most illiterate population such procedure is frustrating. Therefore, they skip government hospitals and approach readily available quacks. On the otherhand, when a hospital has an image and reputation of good service, whether private, or government, patients flock around it. Therefore, the fact that the client needs psychological satisfaction etc., may be kept in mind by the doctors and other staff to make the service satisfactory to them. This can be achieved through better training, effective supervision, utilisation of the findings of studies on various needs of the clients and so on.

PROGRAMMES FOR CHILDREN, PREGNANT MOTHERS AND THE ELDERLY

In our society, children, pregnant mothers and elderly people are handicapped and deserve special consideration in the comprehensive health policy of a welfare state. These people face the risk of morbidity and mortality and their protection remain as a major determinant of success in health and family planning programmes.

There is strong linkage between infant mortality with high fertility. Again there is strong linkage between old age security, value of children and high fertility. Once again better health and social status of mothers influence child survival and success of family planning programme. Therefore, success of health policy and also population control programmes is conditioned by the health care and survival chances assured to children, mothers and the elderly population in a country. Hence, based on the empirical research findings, suitable and effective health promotion programmes may have to be promoted for these three important groups in the population in order to achieve success in the future policy and programmes in the field of health. For details on information in these areas, attention of the readers is drawn to a recent contribution on public health (Pisharoti et al., 1986).

Thus, for the success of health delivery system in India, several new policies and programmes are to be considered beyond the health policy announced by the previous Indian government. In fact that document is not a real policy to meet the growing needs of the population in this field. What is spelt out in the preceding pages also does not cover the entire new thrust of policy formulation for a comprehensive and effective health delivery system for this country. For want of time and space we have highlighted four major issues, viz., (i) Realistic increase in allocation of finance for this programme; (ii) Maximising the use of the existing facilities (iii) Improvement in infrasturctural facilities like worker-population ratio; and (iv) Priority for certain programmes and clients for expanding and succeeding the health delivery system.

For the latter aspects, a few strategies have been discussed, but many more are to be considered on a decentralised manner to meet the diverse needs of population in different regions of the country. A major change needed in existing programme is to make health education compulsory for every body, which is a neglected area though required high priority in the developing countries. In addition, special programmes for the vulnerable group of populations viz., children, pregnant mothers and old people may require immediate attention.

REFERENCES

1. Mahadevan, K. & M. Sumangala, 1987 : Social Development, Cultural Change and Fertility Decline. New Delhi, SAGE International.
2. Mahadevan, K. (Ed.), 1990 : Health Policy, Strategy and Child Survival: Experiences from Asian Countries. D.K. Publishers, New Delhi.
3. Mahadevan, K. et al., 1990 : Family Planning Policies and Strategies for Third World Countries. Paper Presented at Afro-Asian Seminar, June 20-27.
4. Mahadevan, K. (Ed.), 1989 : Fertility Policies in Asian countries. SAGE International, New Delhi.
5. Pisharoti, K.A. et al., 1986 : Education for Better Health of Mother and Child in Primary Health Care. Proceedings of First South East Asian Regional Conference, Madras, 5-8 November.
6. Population Reference Bureau, 1983 : World Population Data Sheet. Washington.
7. Rahimah, Mohd. 1990 : Country Report on Malaysia. Rural Health and Family Planning. Paper presented at the workshop on rural health and family planning, Gandhigram, India 20-26, June.
8. Rosoff, 1989 : Sex education and information. In David, Henry P. United States and Denmark : Different Approaches to Health Care and Family Planning. Studies in Family Planning Vol. 21, No. 1, January/Feb.
9. United Nations, 1989 : Adolescent Reproductive Behaviour : Evidence from Developing Countries, Vol. II, Population Studies No. 109/Add.,/ New Delhi.

INDEX

I

P

Q

R

S

T

U

V

W